RADIOLOGY FOR
DENTAL AUXILIARIES

RADIOLOGY FOR
DENTAL AUXILIARIES

HERBERT H. FROMMER, A.B., D.D.S.

Professor and Director of Radiology,
New York University College of Dentistry,
New York City

THIRD EDITION

With **394** illustrations

The C. V. Mosby Company

ST. LOUIS   TORONTO   1983

MOSBY

A TRADITION OF PUBLISHING EXCELLENCE

Editor: Darlene B. Warfel
Assistant editor: Melba J. Steube
Manuscript editor: Patricia Gayle May
Book design: Jeanne Bush
Cover design: Suzanne Oberholtzer
Production: Barbara Merritt

THIRD EDITION

The C.V. Mosby Company
11830 Westline Industrial Drive, St. Louis, Missouri 63146

Library of Congress Cataloging in Publication Data

Frommer, Herbert H., 1933-
    Radiology for dental auxiliaries.

    Bibliography: p.
    Includes index.
    1. Teeth—Radiography. 2. Dental assistants.
I. Title [DNLM: 1. Dental auxiliaries.
2. Radiography, Dental. WN 230 F932r]
RK309.F76   1983   617.6'07572'024613   82-8123
ISBN 0-8016-1704-9   AACR2

GW/VII/VII 9 8 7 6 5 4 3   02/D/241

To my wife

Ellie

without whose help
this book would not have been possible

Preface

There have been many changes in the field of dental radiology since the first edition of this book was published in 1974. Some of these changes have involved advances in technology, while others have been brought about by forces and events outside the profession. These advances in technology have been accompanied by a heightened public and governmental concern with the use of ionizing radiation. The Three Mile Island incident, disclosures of radiation exposure during atomic testing, and the forces of consumerism have led the public to question the need and the safety of diagnostic radiology in dentistry and medicine.

Could anyone have predicted in 1974 that there would be specific federal legislation enacted that applies to the radiographic practices of dental auxiliaries? The Consumer-Patient Radiation Health and Safety Act of 1981 is just such legislation. It calls for the promulgation of standards for certification of persons who administer radiographic procedures. The bill specifically refers to "dental auxiliaries (including dental hygienists and assistants)" as the group in the dental profession to whom these rules will apply, as dentists are exempt.

The recognized role of the dental auxiliary in radiographic procedures is not being challenged, it is being scrutinized for standards of competency. We of the dental profession must respond to the challenge by maintaining and, in some cases, upgrading our educational and professional standards. Hopefully, this book will aid in the process.

This edition strives, as did the first and second editions, to bridge the gap between basic radiologic principles and clinical competence. Its aim is to instill in dental auxiliaries a respect for the radiation with which they are working. This is a respect for the amount of useful information that can help improve or maintain the dental health of the patient and a respect for the potential harm to patient, auxiliary, and dentist.

Finally, a word of credit and thanks to some of the people whose help and encouragement made my task in preparing this edition much easier; to my colleagues in the Radiology Department of New York University College of Dentistry; Carol Robson for her illustrations; Rosemary Guarino for her preparation of the manuscript; and my wife Eleanor and my sons Ross and Danny for their patience, understanding, and tolerance.

Herbert H. Frommer

Contents

chapter 1   Basic principles of x-ray generation and image production

A preliminary understanding of x-rays and x-ray generation can be acquired by simply visualizing the everyday office routine of handling a patient who needs dental radiographs. The patient is seated in the dental chair and draped with a lead apron, and a film packet is positioned in his mouth. The dental x-ray machine (Fig. 1-1) is turned on by an activating switch and then aimed at the film in the patient's mouth by means of an open-ended cylinder or rectangular position indicating device. The film is exposed by pressing a button attached to an electric cord leading to the x-ray machine. The film is then processed and interpreted by the dentist.

From this description some important observations on the properties of x-rays can be made. X-rays are produced by a machine whose source of energy is electricity: the machine is plugged into an electric outlet and switched on; x-rays are produced by pushing a button that completes an electric circuit. Since during the interval of exposure no sign of x-ray production is apparent, it is established that x-rays are invisible. The x-ray beam is directed at the film packet, so x-rays must travel in straight lines.

The ability of x-rays to produce an image on the film packet inside the patient's mouth by a machine positioned outside the mouth indicates that x-rays can penetrate an opaque structure such as skin or teeth.

After having penetrated the dense tissue, x-rays can produce an effect on a photographic emulsion such as the dental film placed in the patient's mouth. This effect is then made visible by processing the film in the darkroom so that an image of the penetrated structures appears on the film.

Because there are undesirable effects from x-rays, the patient is draped with a lead apron for protection and the operator either leaves the room or stands 6 feet away from the machine when the exposure is made.

To sum up, following are some of the properties of x-rays we have observed:

1. X-rays are produced by the conversion of electric energy.
2. X-rays are invisible.
3. X-rays travel in straight lines.
4. X-rays can penetrate opaque tissues and structures.
5. X-rays can affect a photographic emulsion, which after processing will produce a visible image.
6. X-rays can affect living tissue.

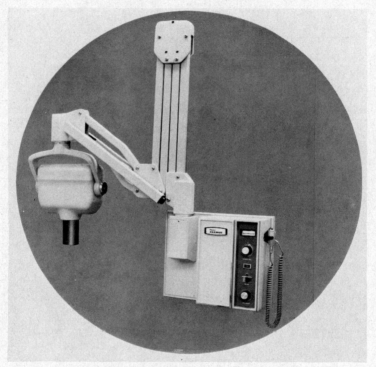

Fig. 1-1. Dental x-ray machine. (Courtesy S.S. White Dental Products International, Pennwalt Corp.)

RADIATION

Radiation is the emission and propagation of energy through space or a substance in the form of waves or particles. Particulate radiation is made of small particles that have mass and usually an electric charge. Some examples of particulate radiation are electrons, sometimes called beta particles, protons, and neutrons. It is with the wave form of radiation that we are most concerned since x-rays are energy waves and are part of a grouping called electromagnetic radiation.

ELECTROMAGNETIC SPECTRUM

The electromagnetic spectrum is a grouping of energy waves that have in common their weightlessness and the speed at which they travel (186,000 miles per second). The individual radiations of the spectrum differ in their wavelength and frequency. Those with the shorter wavelengths and higher frequency have more photon energy.

It is not known whether these electromagnetic radiations are actually waves of energy or individual units of energy called photons. Some phenomena can best be explained using the wave theory and some by considering the theory of discrete units of energy. If the radiation is considered a wave, it is measured by its length. If it is considered a bundle of photon energy, it can be measured in ergs.

Let us consider the concept of an energy wave. An energy wave travels in the same way that a ripple crosses a body of still water. The height of the wave is called the crest, and the depth of the wave is called the trough. The distance from one crest to another is called the wavelength and is usually abbreviated with the Greek letter lambda (λ) (Fig. 1-3). The wavelength of x-rays is very short and is measured in Angstrom units, which are 1/100,000,000 of a centimeter and can be expressed as 10^{-8} cm. The difference in the electromagnetic spectrum between visible light and x-rays is their wavelengths; X-rays have shorter wavelengths. The shorter the wavelength, the more energy it bears, and it is this energy that gives the x-ray the ability to penetrate matter—specifically, the teeth, bones, and gingivae of the dental patient.

In the diagram of the electromagnetic spectrum (see Fig. 1-2) there can be seen energy waves, other than x-rays, with which we are familiar in our daily lives, for example, radio, television, microwave, and electric waves.

The effect of the electromagnetic radiations on living organisms varies depending on their wavelengths. Television waves and radiowaves, which are ever present in the atmosphere, have no effect on human tissue. Microwaves, which are low energy radiations, can produce heat within organic tissues and are so employed in microwave ovens. Microwaves do not have enough energy to be ionizing and therefore do not have the same effects on living tissue as x-rays, gamma rays, or particulate radiations.

3

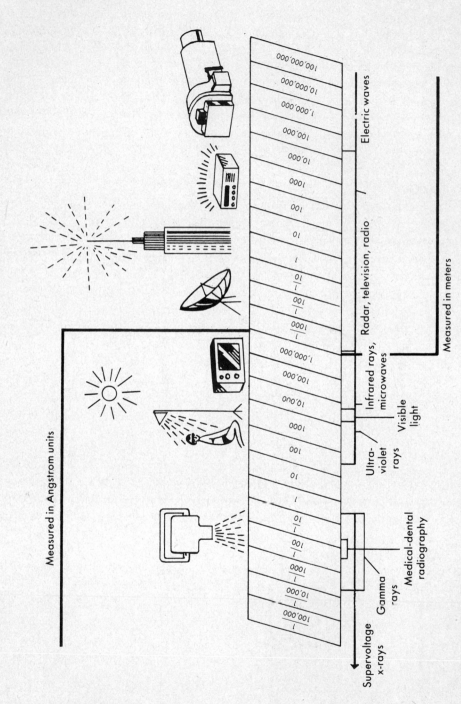

Fig. 1-2. Electromagnetic spectrum. The shorter more energized waves to the left are measured in Angstrom units, the longer waves are measured in meters.

Fig. 1-2 shows that there is an overlap between gamma rays and the x-rays used for diagnostic purposes in medicine and dentistry, because both have identical wavelengths. Gamma rays and x-rays have identical properties; they differ only in their source. X-rays are the result of electron and atomic interaction within an x-ray tube, whereas gamma rays originate within the nucleus of radioactive materials.

To understand the energy aspect of radiation, let us use the example of throwing a ball. In doing this we are imparting energy to the ball, which is expressed by the speed with which the ball travels. As this energy is lost, the ball falls, hits the ground, and rolls to a stop. The total energy is lost when the ball stops. This is also true of radiation. As x-rays travel over a distance, they lose their energy. For this reason, in the dental office the operator stands a safe distance (6 feet) away from the patient being exposed to x-rays to avoid unnecessary exposure.

If the ball is caught in midair the energy can be felt by the impact on the hand catching the moving ball. The impact of the ball is in part a product of the weight of the ball and the speed with which it was thrown. X-rays and other radiations have no weight; they have only speed and energy. But their effect is as tangible as the sting of the ball on the hand. This effect is produced by interaction with the basic unit of matter, the atom.

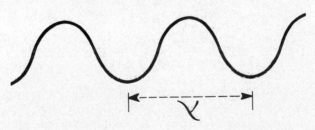

Fig. 1-3. Diagram of x-ray energy wave. The distance between the two crests is the wavelength lambda (λ).

ATOMIC STRUCTURE

All matter is made of atoms. An atom is composed of a relatively heavy inner core or nucleus that possesses a positive electric charge and a number of light, negatively charged particles called electrons that orbit around the nucleus (Fig. 1-4). The nucleus of an atom is composed of positively charged particles called protons and neutral charge particles called neutrons. The number of protons in the nucleus of an element is specific for each element and determines its atomic number. An atom of an element that has the required number of protons but a different number of neutrons in the nucleus is said to be an isotope of the element. Isotopes may be stable or unstable, and the unstable isotopes may give off gamma rays.

In the neutral atom the number of orbiting electrons (−) equals the number of protons (+) in the nucleus; hence, the atom is electrically neutral.

Electrons travel around the nucleus in definite orbits called shells. There is a maximum number of electrons that can occupy each shell and a definite energy level that binds the electrons in each shell to the nucleus. The shells farthest from the nucleus have less binding energy than the inner shells. The shell closest to the nucleus is called the K shell, the next outer shell the L shell, and then successively the M, N, and O shells.

Atoms in turn join to form molecules. A molecule is the smallest particle of a substance that retains the property of the substance.

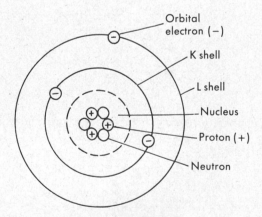

Fig. 1-4. Diagram of an atom. This is a lithium atom whose atomic number (Z) is 3 and its mass number (A) is 6.

IONIZATION

When an orbiting electron is ejected from its shell in an electrically stable or neutral atom, the process is called ionization (Fig. 1-5). The electrically neutral atom has been changed into two ions. The remainder of the atom now has a positive charge and the ejected electron has a negative charge. The energy for this ionization process is the x-ray photon. The new ions do not have all the same properties of the former neutral atom. X-rays as well as gamma rays and some particulate radiation can cause this type of reaction and so are classified as ionizing radiation.

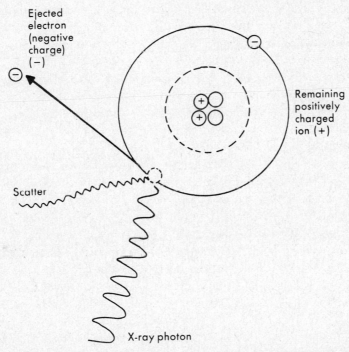

Fig. 1-5. Diagram of ionization. The x-ray photon interacts with a neutral atom to form negatively and positively charged ions.

HISTORY

The x-ray was discovered in November 1895 by Wilhelm Conrad Roentgen, a professor of physics at Wurzberg University in Germany. He was working with a vacuum tube called a Crookes tube, through which an electric current was passed (Fig. 1-6). Roentgen, like many of his colleagues, was interested in the cathode ray produced across the tube when an electric current was applied. Since he was concerned with light, he was working in a darkened room, and there were many fluorescent plates in his laboratory. This was the scene for one of the most important discoveries that would aid medical and dental science.

On the day of the discovery Roentgen noticed that one of the fluorescent plates at the far side of the room was glowing. He quickly realized that something coming from the Crookes tube was striking the fluorescent plate and causing it to glow. Since he did not know what it was, he called the phenomenon x-ray, x being the algebraic designation for the unknown. By placing various objects in the path of the x-ray beam he was able to produce images on the screen. Some of the first radiographs that Roentgen took were of his wife's hand and his shotgun. For his work in the discovery of x-rays, Roentgen received the Nobel Prize in 1901.

Roentgen published his work, and in January 1896 Dr. Otto Walkhoff, a dentist in Braunschweig, Germany, made the first dental use of an x-ray, a radiograph of a lower premolar. He used a small glass photographic plate wrapped in black paper and covered with rubber. The exposure time was 25 minutes. Today, for comparable exposure, we would use about $^3/_{10}$ second.

C. Edmond Kells, a New Orleans dentist, is credited for having taken the first intraoral radiographs in 1896. Other early workers with intraoral radiographs were W.J. Morton and William Rollins. It was Rollins who developed the first dental x-ray unit in 1896.

Many of the early workers with dental x-rays suffered from effects of their work. William Rollins reported burns to the skin of his hands and C. Edmond Kells, before his death, had three fingers, his hand, and, finally, his arm amputated. Dr. Kells used a technique called "setting the tube" to adjust the x-ray beam. He held his hand between the tube and a fluoroscope and adjusted the beam quality until the bones of his hand were seen clearly.

In 1913, William D. Coolidge invented the hot cathode x-ray tube, which is the prototype of x-ray tubes used today. The hot filament provided a variable source of electrons in the tube and eliminated the need for residual gas as a source for ionization in the tube.

It was also in 1913 that the first American dental x-ray machine was manufactured. In 1923, the Victor X-ray Corporation, which later became General Electric X-ray Corporation, introduced a dental x-ray machine with a Coolidge tube in the head of the unit cooled by oil immersion.

The x-rays were produced in Roentgen's vacuum tube because the electric current applied to the tube caused ionization of the gas molecules in the tube. That is, the neutral molecules were broken up into negative ions and positive ions. Because of the difference in electric potential, the negative particles (electrons) were attracted to the positive side of the tube where they collided with the tube wall, and x-rays were produced. Modern dental x-ray tubes employ the same principle with some modifications, the most significant being a higher voltage or difference in potential across the tube and a variable source of electrons (hot filament) plus radiation safety features and cooling devices.

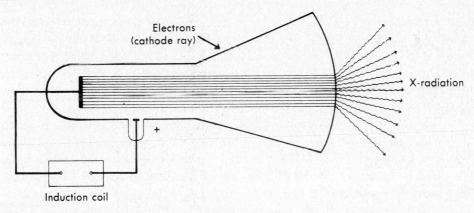

Fig. 1-6. Crookes tube, which Roentgen worked with at the time of the discovery of x-rays in 1895.

ELECTRICITY

Since the primary source of energy for the x-ray machine is electricity, it is necessary to learn or review some basic concepts of electricity.

Electric current is the flow of electricity through a circuit; it can either be alternating (AC) or direct (DC). By direct current we mean current that flows in only one direction in an electric circuit, whereas alternating current flows in one direction and then flows in the opposite direction in the circuit (Fig. 1-7). The term *cycle* in alternating current refers to the flow of current in one direction and then the reversal and flowing of the current in the opposite direction. There are usually 60 cycles per second in most alternating current circuits.

Voltage is the term used to describe the electric potential or force that drives an electric current through a circuit. The unit of measurement is the volt. The kilovolt (kV) is 1000 volts. In an alternating current, where the direction of the current is constantly changing, the voltage is also changing, and the term *kilovolt peak* (kVp) is used to denote the maximum or peak voltage that is described by the sine wave that plots the alternation of the current (see Fig. 1-7). A dental x-ray machine that is set for a potential of 90 kV will only reach 90 kV at the peak of the alternating current during exposure. As seen in the diagram of the exposure's sine wave, other voltage levels also occur during the exposure. This has great clinical significance because these differences in voltage contribute to the heterogeneity of the x-ray beam.

Ampere is the unit of measurement used to describe the amount of electric current flowing through a circuit. The millampere (mA) is equal to $1/1000$ of an ampere.

A *transformer* is a device that can either increase or decrease the voltage in an electric circuit. It is composed of two coils of electric wire insulated from one another. The magnetic field from one coil induces an electric current in the second coil. The number of turns in the induction coil in relation to the number of turns in the second coil will determine what the action of the transformer will be. The dental x-ray machine also has an *autotransformer,* which utilizes only one coil and can be used only for making minor changes in voltage. If the transformer increases the voltage, it is referred to as a "step-up" transformer, and if it decreases the voltage, it is referred to as a "step-down" transformer. The dental x-ray machine utilizes both types in taking ordinary line or house voltage of 110 volts and stepping it up to a range of 65,000 to 100,000 volts (65 to 100 kVp) in the high tension circuit, or stepping line voltage down to 3 to 5 volts in the filament circuit, these being the two basic circuits in the dental x-ray machine.

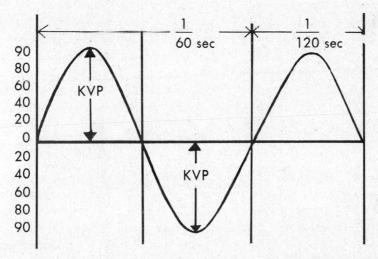

Fig. 1-7. Sine wave of 60-cycle electric current operating at 90,000 volts (90 kVp).

THE DENTAL X-RAY MACHINE

Control panel (Fig. 1-8)

The control panel of the dental x-ray machine contains an on-off switch and indicator light, an exposure button and indicator light, timer dial, kVp and mA selectors. The exposure button is on a 6-foot retractable cord or linked to a remote station. Some machines have preset fixed milliamperage choices, usually 10 or 15 mA or both. The kVp values may be fixed or have a range from 65 to 100.

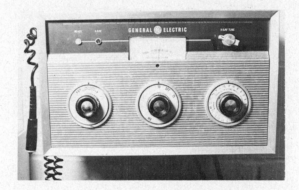

Fig. 1-8. Control panel of dental x-ray machine.

Circuitry (Fig. 1-9)

Dental x-ray machines use 110-volt alternating current. There are two major circuits in the x-ray machine, the filament circuit and the high voltage circuit. Each circuit utilizes a transformer to convert the line voltage and current. The filament circuit uses 3 to 5 volts and so the 110 volt line current is reduced by means of a step-down transformer. The heating of the cathode filament by the electric current is controlled by a rheostat in the circuit and is a function of the millamperage selector on the control panel of the machine. The high voltage circuit in the dental x-ray machine requires voltage in the range of 65,000 to 100,000 volts. This increase in voltage is achieved by the use of a step-up transformer. An autotransformer is also used in the circuit as a line compensator to control fluctuations in line voltage. The relationship of the input circuit to a variable number of coils is changed in the autotransformer, by the kVp dial on the control panel, to change the quality of the x-rays emitted.

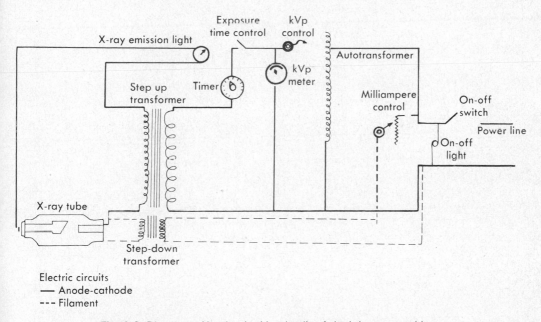

Fig. 1-9. Diagram of basic electric circuits of dental x-ray machine.

The x-ray tube

The dental x-ray tube, housed in a large machine, is about 6 inches long and 1½ inches in diameter.

The three basic elements of an x-ray tube needed to produce x-rays are: (1) high voltage to accelerate electrons across the tube, (2) a source of electrons within the tube, and (3) a target to stop the electrons.

High voltage. As we can see in Fig. 1-10, the x-ray tube has a positive side (pole) called the anode and a negative side called the cathode. Electric current flows from a negative pole to a positive pole. This voltage can be varied by adjusting the kilovoltage dial found on the dental x-ray machine control panel. It is the kilovoltage dial that actually controls the autotransformer, which then affects the step-up transformer and thus the kilovoltage across the tube. The greater the kilovoltage or potential across the tube, the faster the electrons will travel and the greater the energy that will be released when the electrons strike the target at the anode.

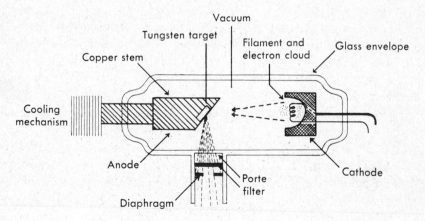

Fig. 1-10. Components of a dental x-ray tube.

Source of electrons. The main source of electrons in the x-ray tube is the tungsten filament found at the cathode. This is a variable source of electrons, unlike Roentgen's tube in which electrons were produced from the ionization of a fixed volume of gas. The tungsten filament is connected to the step-down transformer circuit. The hotter the resistant filament becomes, the more electrons that are produced at the cathode. This production, or boiling off, of electrons from the heated tungsten filament is called the *thermionic emission effect*. The milliamperage dial controls the amount of current in the filament circuit and hence the number of electrons that "boil off." The tungsten filament is surrounded by the molybdenum focusing cup, which directs electrons toward the anode that contains the target.

The target. The target in the x-ray tube can also be called the focal spot or area. It is at the anode part of the tube, and when the circuit is complete, it has a positive (+) charge. It is made of tungsten and measures about 0.8×1.8 mm. This is the actual target. The effective target or focal area is smaller because of the tilting of the target that geometrically makes the target smaller when viewed from the opening in the tube. All modern dental x-ray machines have approximately the same size target. Tungsten is used as the target material because it has a high melting point and a low vapor pressure at high temperatures and thus will not be affected by the heat produced. The element tungsten is also desirable as a target material because of its high atomic number, and thus its density, and because when it is bombarded by electrons, x-ray production is more efficient. Tungsten, however, does not have a high degree of thermal conductivity and must be imbedded in a copper stem. The heat is dissipated into the head of the x-ray machine by the copper stem attached to the anode and cooled by air or oil immersion.

Timer. The dental x-ray tube does not emit a continuous stream of radiation but rather a series of impulses of radiation. The number of impulses depends on the number of cycles per second in the electric current being used. In 60-cycle alternating current, there are 60 pulses of x-ray per second. Each impulse lasts only $1/120$ second since no x-rays are emitted in the negative half of the cycle when the polarity of the tube is reversed. The newer model dental x-ray machine exposure dials are not calibrated in fractions of seconds, but more realistically in impulses. On the timer dial "24" means 24 impulses per second, which is equivalent to a $2/5$-$(24/60)$ second exposure. With the advent of more sensitive or faster films calling for decreased exposure times, all machines should have electronically controlled timers so that these short exposure times can be achieved accurately and repetitively. The old mechanical timers with increments of $1/4$ second, which were usually at least $1/8$ to $1/4$ second inaccurate, are unacceptable for the shorter exposure times in use.

Tube position. Until recently, the x-ray tube was placed in the anterior part of the head of the machine close to the position indicating device or "cone" (Fig. 1-11). The rest of the head of the x-ray machine contained electric circuitry and cooling devices. The cone or open-ended cylinder, properly referred to as a "position indicating device" (PID), placed on the head of the machine, served as the aiming device for the x-ray beam and the length of this cone determined the focal distance to be used. There was objection to the long cones as being bulky, cumbersome, and difficult to operate in small operatories. It was also said that the long cone tended to unbalance the head of the x-ray machine. With the increasing popularity of the paralleling technique and the need for an extended focal-film distance, a new design for tube heads was introduced by one of the leading manufacturers.

It can be seen in Fig. 1-11 how the new design operates. The x-ray tube is placed in the rear part of the head of the machine and the rest of the components are placed on both sides of the beam. The advantage of the design is found in the extended focal distance and the elimination of the long bulky cone. The terms "short" and "long" cone are no longer appropriate. Cones are now outdated because of radiation hygiene, having been replaced by open-ended lead-lined cylinders and rectangles and also because the machine with the "short cone" may really have a "long" focal-film distance, depending on the placement of the x-ray tube in the head of the machine.

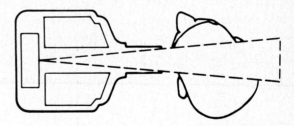

Fig. 1-11. Long beam tube head *(top)* and conventional tube head *(bottom)*. Note different position of x-ray tube itself that allows for increased focal film distance. (Courtesy S.S. White Dental Products International, Pennwalt Corp.)

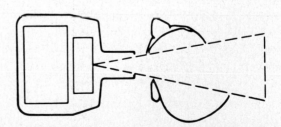

CLOSED CONE vs OPEN CYLINDER OR RECTANGULAR DEVICES

Since we have been discussing cone and cylinder length, let us now turn our attention to the open-ended PID as opposed to the closed and pointed cone. The pointed cone was designed as an easy aiming device, the tip of the cone indicating the position of the central ray. The technique called for aiming the tip of the cone at the center of the film packet placed in the patient's mouth or the extraoral anatomic landmark being used. One of the unfortunate outcomes of this type of instrumentation was that some practitioners came to believe that the x-ray beam was coming out only from the tip of the cone.

The problem with the pointed plastic cone is the secondary radiation that is produced by the interaction of the primary beam of x-ray photons with the plastic cone (Fig. 1-12). These secondary x-rays increase the long wavelength radiation to the patient's face and degrade the diagnostic image on the film. X-rays do interact with plastic even though one might not consider it to be a very dense material. X-rays will interact and cause secondary radiation with any form of matter from a piece of tissue paper to a bar of steel. The density of the material and the quality of the x-ray beam determine the type and extent of interaction. When the open-ended PID is used there is no material at the end of the PID with which to interact. Some practitioners have complained about the open-ended PIDs, claiming that they are difficult to aim properly and that cone cutting results. In reality, it is not that the cylinder is difficult to use but that the change from the pointed cone is difficult to make. Novice dental students starting instruction in radiology have no more difficulty using the open-ended PIDs than their predecessors had with the pointed cone.

Radiation protection codes in many states have mandated the use of the open-ended cylinder. It is strongly recommended that the use of pointed cones be terminated and open-ended lead-lined cylinders or rectangular devices be used instead.

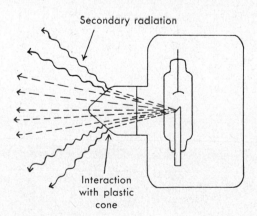

Secondary radiation

Interaction
with plastic
cone

Fig. 1-12. Production of secondary radiation resulting from interaction of the primary beam with the closed-end plastic cone.

X-RAY PRODUCTION

When a dental x-ray machine is turned on and the indicator light is glowing, it is ready to produce x-rays. The turning on of the machine completes the filament circuit and heats the tungsten filament. The electrons stay at the filament in what is called the electron cloud (Fig. 1-13). The electrons will be attracted across the tube only when there is a difference in electric potential or, stated another way, when the high-voltage circuit is completed. This high-voltage circuit is activated by the exposure switch and remains active for the length of time for which a timer is set.

With the high-voltage circuit completed by closing of the exposure switch, the electrons produced by the thermionic emission effect at the cathode are attracted to the positively charged anode (Fig. 1-14). This stream of electrons crossing the tube is called the cathode ray.

Recently enacted federal regulations regarding new dental x-ray machines require that an audible signal be sounded when an exposure is being made, in addition to the signal lights in the control panel.[1]

X-rays as well as heat are produced in the tube when the high speed electrons strike the tungsten target (Fig. 1-15). This is a transference of energy. The kinetic energy of the moving electron is converted into the energy laden x-ray photon and heat energy. The faster the electrons travel across the tube, the more energized and penetrating will be the x-rays produced. The speed of the electrons across the tube is determined by the kilovoltage.

As illustrated in Fig. 1-10 the tungsten target is angled and the x-rays produced are directed to an exit point (porte) in the tube. The rest of the x-ray tube is lead-lined, and it is only through the porte that x-rays can leave the tube. If x-rays leave the tube in any area other than the porte, the machine is said to have lead leakage. This is a safety hazard to both patient and operator.

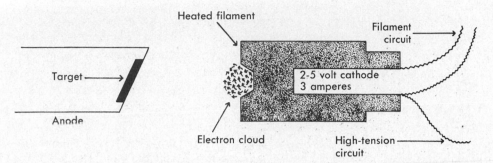

Fig. 1-13. An x-ray tube illustrating formation of an electron cloud at the cathode as filament circuit is activated.

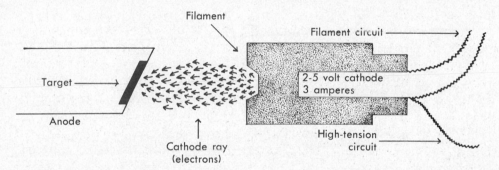

Fig. 1-14. An x-ray tube showing electrons traveling across the tube from the cathode to anode (target) as high-tension circuit (exposure switch) is activated.

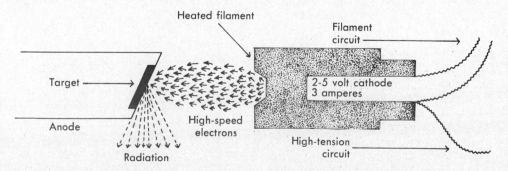

Fig. 1-15. An x-ray tube showing production of x-rays as high-speed electrons collide with target.

Bremsstrahlung and characteristic x-rays

The phenomenon of x-ray production can be best understood by considering the tungsten atom and the possibilities that arise when a high speed electron enters its orbit as it would at the target of a dental x-ray machine (Fig. 1-16). The tungsten target is made up of an infinite number of tungsten atoms. We will consider only one surface atom that will serve as a representative example for the rest of the atoms in the tungsten target.

The first possibility, which rarely occurs, is that the high speed electron might hit the nucleus of the tungsten atom and give up all its energy. The second possibility is that the high speed electron might hit and dislodge one of the orbiting electrons of the tungsten atom. This can happen only when the entering electrons possess more energy than that binding the orbiting electrons to the nucleus. In the dental machine this means it can happen only at settings of 70 kVp and above because the binding energy of the K shell of electrons is 69,000 electron volts. If an orbiting electron is dislodged, there is a rearrangement or cascading of electrons inward to fill up the electron vacancies in the inner shells. This rearrangement produces a loss of energy that is expressed in x-ray

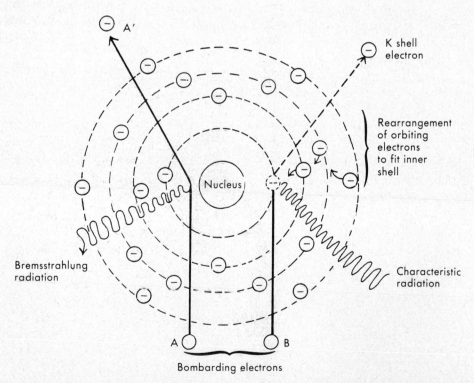

Fig. 1-16. Electrons colliding with simulated tungsten atom. Forming *a*, Bremsstrahlung radiation, and *b*, characteristic radiation.

energy. The x-rays thus produced are called characteristic x-rays and account for a very small part of the x-rays produced in the dental machine and only in those machines operating at 70 kVp and above. The third possibility is that the entering high speed electron might be slowed down and bent off its course by the positive pull of the nucleus. This slowing down represents a loss of energy that is given off as x-rays and heat.

The major source of x-ray production in the dental x-ray tube is the last possibility. The slowing down and veering off course of the high speed entering electron with its loss of energy expressed in x-rays and heat is called bremsstrahlung. This is the German word for "breaking radiation."

Heat production

It must be pointed out that the dental x-ray machine is an extremely inefficient machine. That is, of the total energy produced at the anode by the collision of the electrons with the target, less than 1% is x-ray energy; the remaining 99% is in the form of heat. This is the reason for the highly conductive copper sleeve and oil immersion tube surrounding the target. Care must be taken not to overheat the tube.

Under ordinary use, overheating of a dental x-ray machine is not very likely. Each machine has a duty rating and a duty cycle. The duty rating refers to the number of consecutive seconds a machine can be operated before overheating, and the duty cycle refers to the portion of every minute that a dental machine can be used without overheating.

Rectification

The previous discussion has failed to take into account that in almost all cases the dental x-ray machine is operating on alternating current. This means that in the x-ray tube itself the polarity is reversed 60 times per second. When the direction of the current flow is reversed, the tungsten target becomes the negative pole or cathode and the tungsten filament becomes the positive pole or anode. During the alternating $1/120$ second ($\frac{1}{2}$ cycle) when the current is reversed, no x-rays are produced, for there are no electrons at the target available to travel across the tube and strike the target, and so the current is blocked from traveling across the tube. This blocking of the reversal is called rectification, and since the dental x-ray tube does this because of its own design, it is said to be self-rectified.

So we see that x-rays are not produced in a steady stream but in spurts or pulses and that these pulses take place only during one half of the alternating current cycle. Since most alternating current is 60 cycles, the dental x-ray machines will express exposure units in pulses or sixtieths of a second instead of the usual $\frac{1}{2}$ second or $3/10$ second. A $\frac{1}{2}$ second exposure is equal to 30 pulses. It should be obvious that exposure time of $3/7$ second is not possible, since it is not divisible into 60, and it is impossible to get a fraction of a cycle of alternating current.

21

X-RAY BEAM

The x-ray photons produced at the target in the dental x-ray tube emanate as a divergent beam. The x-ray at the center of the beam is referred to as the central ray. The x-rays closest to the central ray will be more parallel and those farthest away more divergent. It is the more parallel rays that will produce less magnification of the image (Fig. 1-17).

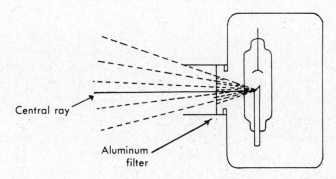

Fig. 1-17. The divergent x-ray beam. The aluminum filter removes longer wavelength x-rays from the beam.

Interaction of x-rays with matter

X-rays interact with all forms of matter. This interaction can result in absorption of energy (a reduction of the intensity of the x-ray beam) and the production of secondary radiation.

Primary radiation is the result of the x-rays produced at the target of the anode in the x-ray tube. Secondary radiation is the result of the interaction of primary radiation with matter (see Fig. 2-4).

When x-rays are absorbed by matter, positive and negative ions, as well as secondary radiation, are formed from previously neutral molecules. The amount and type of absorption that takes place depend on the energy of the x-ray beam (the wavelength) and the composition of the absorbing matter. The thicker the material that an x-ray beam has to penetrate, the more x-rays that will be absorbed. It is, however, not just thickness that determines x-ray absorption. The atomic configuration—the number of orbiting electrons, protons, and neutrons in the nucleus of the atom—also determine x-ray absorption. Heavy elements, those with greater mass, are better absorbers than lighter elements. The more electrons available in an absorbing material, the more x-ray photons that are absorbed. Heavy metals with high atomic numbers (the atomic number indicates the number of protons and electrons in an atom), such as lead and gold, absorb x-rays readily.

An important point to be made is that when x-rays are absorbed by any material, that material does not become radioactive because x-rays have no effect on the nucleus of the absorbing atom. This means that the equipment or walls in a dental operatory do not become radioactive after continuous exposure to radiation. At the atomic level there are four possibilities that can occur when an x-ray photon interacts with matter. These possibilities are:

1. No interaction (pass through). The x-ray photon can pass through the atom unchanged and leave the atom unchanged (Fig. 1-18, A).
2. Thompson scatter (unmodified or coherent scatter). The x-ray photon can have its path altered by the atom. There is no change to the absorbing atom but a photon of scattered radiation is produced (Fig. 1-18, A).
3. Photoelectric effect. The x-ray photon can collide with an orbiting electron giving up all its energy to dislodge the electron from its orbit. The photoelectron that is produced will have a negative charge while the remaining atom will have a positive charge. This, you will remember, is ionization (Fig. 1-18, B).
4. Compton effect. The x-ray photon can collide with a loosely bound electron in an outer shell of the atom and only give up part of its energy in ejecting the electron from its orbit. This results in a negatively charged, ejected Compton electron, a photon of scattered radiation, and a remaining atom that is now positively charged. This again is ionization (Fig. 1-18, C).

The Compton and Photoelectric effects are the types of interaction seen with dental x-rays.

23

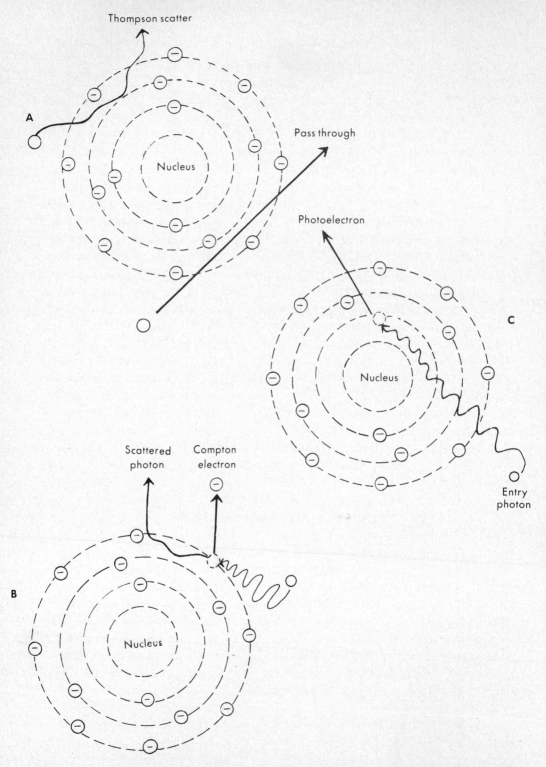

Fig. 1-18. Interaction of x-rays with matter. **A,** Pass through and Thompson scatter. **B,** Photoelectric effect. **C,** Compton effect.

Quality and quantity of x-rays: milliamperage and kilovoltage

The three parameters of the dental x-ray beam that are adjusted from the control panel by either the dental auxiliary or the dentist are the energy, or penetrating power (quality), of the x-ray beam, the number of x-rays produced (quantity), and the length of time that these x-rays will be produced.

Quality. The quality, or penetrating power, of the x-ray beam is controlled by the kilovoltage. The suitable range for dental radiography is 65 to 100 kVp. Some units can deliver this complete range, whereas others have more limited ranges or even a fixed kVp value. As a rule, the kilovoltage in a dental office will remain fixed at one setting for all intraoral radiography. The dentist will determine what kilovoltage will produce the most diagnostic radiographs for the particular use of that office.

Dental diagnostic radiology is confined to the 65 to 100 kVp range because the density of the structures dentistry deals with (teeth, bone, etc.) determines the useful penetration range. Kilovoltage settings below 65 would not give proper penetration of the object without undue production of secondary x-radiation, and kilovoltage above 100 causes overpenetration. The overall objective of diagnostic radiology is to record differences in densities on the films of the objects being radiographed. A kilovoltage range is chosen that will indicate the difference of penetration and absorption so that the differences in structural densities can be recorded. The choice of kVp setting will be discussed in the section on density and contrast. We see, then, that a kilovoltage is selected that will allow for complete absorption of some x-rays, partial absorption of others, and passage of other x-rays through the object.

The radiograph is produced because of differential absorption of the x-ray beam by the object being radiographed. That is why less dense structures, such as the dental pulp, will appear radiolucent (black) on the dental film, and highly calcified denser structures, such as the enamel, will appear radiopaque (white or gray). The less dense areas in the object allow greater passage of x-rays than do denser areas, and more x-rays strike the film in these areas to darken it.

Low kilovoltage rated x-ray machines in the 45 to 65 kVp range are no longer considered acceptable as the radiation produced contains many long nonpenetrating wavelengths that increase the facial exposure to the patient unnecessarily.

Half value layer. The term *half value layer* (HVL) is used to describe beam quality and penetration rather than kilovoltage. Kilovoltage is a description of the electric energy put into an x-ray tube. HVL measures the quality of the x-rays emitted from the tube. Two similar x-ray machines operating at the same kilovoltage may not produce x-rays of the same penetration. The HVL is defined as the thickness of aluminum (measured in millimeters) that will reduce the intensity of the x-ray beam by 50%.

Quantity. The milliampere dial determines the number of x-rays produced in a given exposure time period by controlling the heating of the tungsten filament at the cath-

25

ode of the tube. As the kilovoltage determines the quality (penetrating power) of the x-rays produced, the milliamperage determines the quantity of x-rays produced.

It is better to consider the concept of milliampere seconds (mAs) than milliamperage alone. An exposure at a given kVp of 1 second using 10 mA is 10 mAs. A 2 second exposure at the same kVp using 5 mA would produce an identical film since the mAs are again 10 ($10 \times 1 = 10$, $5 \times 2 = 10$).

The sensitivity of the film used determines the mAs required at a given kilovoltage. The more sensitive the film to radiation, the fewer milliampere seconds required. The advantage of higher milliamperage is that a shorter exposure time can be used. This does not represent a decrease in the patient's x-ray exposure, only a decrease in the time necessary to expose the film. This reduces the chance of blurring caused by patient motion.

Ideally, it would be best to use the shortest exposure time and a high milliamperage to achieve the desired mAs. The range of milliamperage on dental x-ray machines is usually from 5 to 15 mA. The limiting factor is the heat produced at the desired small target. Milliamperage higher than 15 would produce too many electrons bombarding the target, and thus too much heat.

Filtration. The x-ray beam that originates at the anode is not homogeneous. It consists of a spectrum of long and short wavelengths. In fact, very few of the x-ray photons produced have energy or penetration power corresponding to the desired kilovoltage called for on the control panel. In other words, if one sets the kVp dial for any desired kilovoltage, only a few of the x-ray photons produced will correspond to this setting. Almost all the x-ray photons produced will have wavelengths longer than those corresponding to the desired setting and thus, be less penetrating. This is partially due to the electrons in the tube bombarding multiple atomic layers of the tungsten target with the resulting bremsstrahlung and characteristic x-ray production and the effect of alternating current with its sine wave voltage buildup. As we can see in Fig. 1-19, the x-ray beam is not homogeneous but rather heterogeneous, having a full range of wavelengths. The longer, lower, kVp wavelengths will not penetrate tooth and bone and will only be absorbed by the skin or produce secondary radiation.

The function of the filter is to remove from the primary beam the long nonpenetrating wavelength x-rays (see Fig. 1-17). After the primary beam has been filtered and collimated, it is referred to as the useful beam.

Federal regulations require that for dental x ray machines operating at kilovoltages up to 70 kVp, 2 mm of aluminum filtration is required.[1] For those machines operating from 70 kVp and higher, 2.5 mm of aluminum filtration is required.

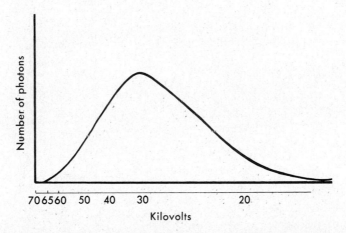

Fig. 1-19. Graph of spectrum of x-ray beam from dental x-ray machine operating at 65 kVp. Note number of low-energy photons produced.

Collimation

The size and shape of the x-ray beam as it leaves the tube head are restricted by a collimating device (Fig. 1-20). In intraoral radiography, the size of the beam must be just large enough to cover the film packet and allow for a slight margin of error in positioning (Fig. 1-21). A beam size any larger than this would expose the patient's face to unnecessary primary radiation. The collimating device most often used is a lead diaphragm with a circular aperture (Fig. 1-22). The size of this aperture, at a selected focal-film distance, determines the beam size. PIDs, be they open-ended cylinders or rectangles, lead-lined or made of metal, can also serve as collimating devices. Federal regulations presently require that the x-ray beam should not exceed 2¾ inches in diameter when measured at the patient's skin.[1]

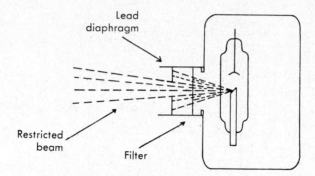

Fig. 1-20. Collimation and filtration of x-ray beam.

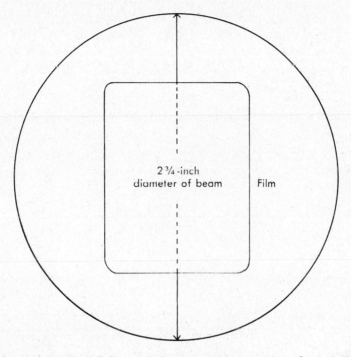

2 ¾ -inch
diameter of beam   Film

Fig. 1-21. Relative size of adult film packet compared to x-ray beam 2¾ inches in diameter.

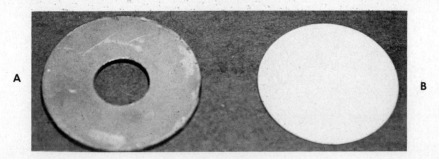

A   B

Fig. 1-22. A, Lead diaphragm. **B,** An aluminum filter.

Rectangular collimation. The shape of the dental x-ray beam has always been circular. The question can be asked, "Why is a circular beam used when the film packet is rectangular in shape?" The circular beam covers a greater facial area, and it exposes the patient to more primary radiation than a tightly collimated rectangular beam does. The movement in the dental profession in now toward rectangular collimation. This change to rectangular collimation can be accomplished without an increase in "cone cutting" with the use of proper equipment. X-ray beam film alignment is easily done by using the "Precision Device" (Isaac Masel Co.) (Fig. 1-23) or the "XCP" (Rinn Corp.) and a metal rectangular PID (Fig. 1-24).

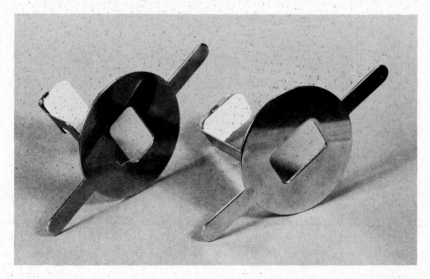

Fig. 1-23. Rectangular collimating device. (Courtesy Precision Instruments, Isaac Masel Co., Inc., Philadelphia.)

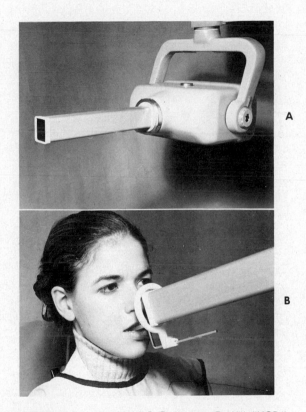

Fig. 1-24. A, Rectangular PID Collimator. **B,** With "XCP."

FACTORS INFLUENCING IMAGE FORMATION

In making radiographs of dental structures, we are striving for a film image with the proper degree of density and contrast, detail sharpness, and a minimum amount of enlargement and distortion.

Density and contrast

Density is the degree of blackness on a film and contrast is the difference in the degrees of blackness between adjacent areas. The density of a film is determined by the relative transmissions of the x-rays by various parts of the object and by the absorption of the x-rays in the emulsion of the film. These two factors, the object being radiographed (object contrast) and the properties of the film (film contrast) determine the overall density and contrast of the finished radiograph.

Object contrast. The object contrast is determined by (1) the thickness of the object, (2) the density of the object, (3) the chemical composition of the object, (4) the quality of the x-ray beam, and (5) scatter radiation. We cannot control the thickness, density, or atomic number of the structures being radiographed. The only variables are quality or penetration of the x-rays (65 or 90 kVp) and the amount of scatter radiation produced.

By varying the kilovoltage and thus the quality of the radiation, either high or low contrast films can be produced.

Short scale. High contrast films appear mainly black and white with very few gray tones. They are also referred to as short scale contrast films and are produced by kilovoltage in the 50 to 65 kVp range. These films are said to be "crisper" and more pleasing to the eye but they may not reveal early pathologic changes. The short scale film is a "yes" or "no" situation: either the x-ray beam penetrates the object or it does not. Areas appear black or white, radiolucent or radiopaque, with few gray tones in the middle range (Fig. 1-25). As mentioned, the lower kVp ratings (below 65) are undesirable as they result in increased facial absorption and scatter because of their less penetrating wavelengths.

Long scale. The low contrast films, also referred to as long scale contrast, are produced by the high kilovoltage range of 90 to 100 kVp. In these films there are many tones of gray in addition to the blacks and whites. The long scale film is not as visually pleasing as the short scale but early changes in object density may be seen in the gradation of the gray tones, which are not present in the high contrast films.

One could choose a kVp in the middle range (70 to 75 kVp) and try to gain some advantage from both techniques.

Scattered radiation produces a uniform exposure over the film and in doing so reduces the contrast. This is referred to as "film fog" and it degrades the diagnostic image. Most scattered radiation originates in the object itself; thus, the larger the field (as in extraoral radiography), the more scatter becomes a factor. In intraoral radiography backscatter

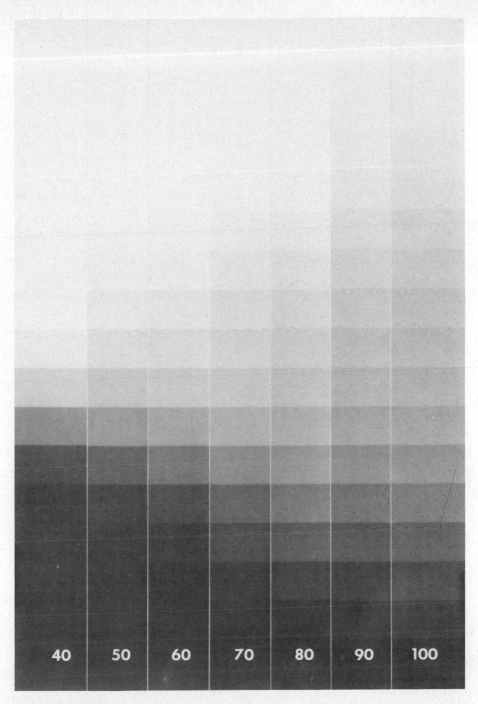

Fig. 1-25. Aluminum step wedge densities. A step wedge of aluminum is radiographed using increasing kVp (penetration). At the thinner portion of the step wedge there is complete penetration at all kVps. At the thicker portion of the wedge, the lower kVp will not penetrate while the higher kVp will penetrate as shown by the gray tones. (Courtesy Eastman Kodak Co.)

is reduced by using as small a beam as possible, open-ended PIDs, and lead backing in the film package.

Film contrast. Film contrast is determined by (1) the amount of radiation transmitted (object contrast), (2) the type of film, (3) intensifying screens, if used, and (4) film processing. Each of these factors is discussed in their respective sections. The important fact is that any secondary radiation or light that affects the film will decrease the desired contrast or "fog" the film, which will degrade the image.

Focal-film distance (FFD) and object-film distance (OFD)

The ideal radiograph of an object, such as a tooth, in regard to definition, image enlargement, and distortion, can be made by meeting the following criteria:

1. Have a maximum focal-film distance (FFD). FFD is the distance between the focal spot (target) at the anode and the film in the patient's mouth. The maximum distance will enable the more parallel rays from the middle of the x-ray beam to strike the object, and not the more divergent x-rays from the periphery of the beam, which would cause image enlargement on the film (Fig. 1-26).
2. Have a minimum object-film distance (OFD). The tooth and the film should be be as close together as possible. The closer they are, the less the enlargement of the image on the film (Fig. 1-26).
3. Have the object and the film parallel to each other in their long axes and the central ray perpendicular to both.

These are the optimum requirements. In intraoral radiography, it is impossible to meet all of these requirements at the same time.

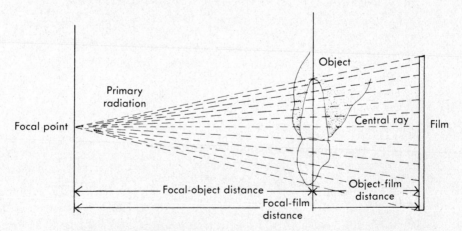

Fig. 1-26. Relationship between focal point, object, and film.

Focal-film distance (FFD). The most common focal-film distances (FFDs) used in dentistry are 8, 12, and 16 inches. An FFD of less than 8 inches may cause magnification of the image that is larger than the film (Fig. 1-27). As the FFD is increased to 12 or 16 inches, the magnification of the image decreases because the image is being formed by the more parallel x-rays from the center of the bundle. However, this decrease in magnification is not a linear relationship beyond 16 inches. As the Fig. 1-28 shows, as the FFD is increased beyond 16 inches, the percentage of magnification does not decrease significantly. Therefore, using a 24 inch FFD does not give a clinically significant better image than a 16-inch FFD. That is why in intraoral radiography, an FFD between 8 and 16 inches is used.

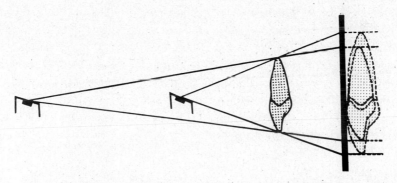

Fig. 1-27. Comparison of 8-inch and 16-inch focal-film distance. (Courtesy Rinn Corp., Elgin, Ill.)

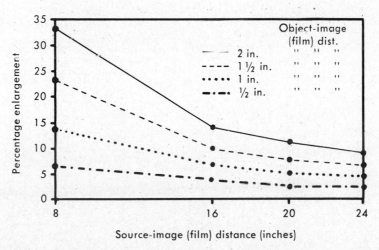

Fig. 1-28. Relationship of image magnification to object-film distance and focal-film distance. (Courtesy Rinn Corp., Elgin, Ill.)

Inverse square law. One of the factors that must be considered when choosing or changing an FFD is the inverse square law. It states that the intensity of radiation varies inversely with the square of the distance. More simply stated, if the FFD is doubled, the exposure time is quadrupled. This assumes that the mA and kVp will remain the same.

Before the advent of the more sensitive films, the inverse square law presented more of a limiting factor than it does today. For instance, if one were using an 8-inch FFD at 1-second exposure and then changed to a 16-inch FFD, a 4-second exposure time would be necessary to produce a comparable film at the same mA and kVp. This 4-second exposure time would be inordinately long and there could be patient movement. With the use of faster x-ray film and exposure times in the range of $^2/_{10}$ second at an 8-inch FFD, a 16-inch FFD would need only $^8/_{10}$-second exposure time. Clinically, $^8/_{10}$-second exposure time, when compared to $^2/_{10}$-second, presents no more or less problem with patient movement. The same amount of radiation is reaching the film in the 8- and 16-inch techniques; it just takes greater time to achieve required x-ray intensity with the increased distance.

Another clinical application of the inverse square law is the positioning of the open-ended cylinder almost touching the patient's face when taking intraoral radiographs. This will give the desired FFD, depending on the length of the PID. If the operator is careless in placement and does not approximate the skin, this will produce an increased FFD and decreased intensity of the x-ray beam by a factor of the square of the distance from the patient's face. A small distance, when squared, can lead to an underexposed film. Most dental offices will select an FFD and keep this technique constant.

Object-film distance (OFD). Because of the anatomy of the mouth it is impossible to satisfy ideal criteria 2 and 3 above, which refer to object-film distance (OFD) and parallelism between the object and the film. If the film is held close to the teeth, then the parallelism will be lost, and if the teeth and film are to be parallel, there must be increased OFD.

This is the basis for the two techniques used in film placement for intraoral radiography: the paralleling technique and the bisecting-angle technique. The details of performing both these techniques, as well as their advantages and disadvantages, will be described in Chapters 3 and 4.

In the paralleling techinque, the film is held parallel to the long axis of the tooth. This results in an increased OFD in most areas of the mouth. That is, for the film to remain parallel to the tooth it must be positioned away from the tooth (Fig. 1-29). The enlargement caused by the increased OFD is compensated for by using an increased FFD (12 or 16 inches). The use of the increased FFD is the reason for the misnomer "long cone technique." It is not the long cone that is of primary importance but the parallelism between the tooth and the film.

In the bisecting-angle technique, the film is held as close to the tooth as possible. At this point the long axis of the tooth and the plane of the film cannot be parallel. A geometric trick is then used to project the proper image of the tooth onto the film. An imaginary line is drawn that bisects the angle formed by the long axis of the tooth and the plane of the dental film (Fig. 1-30). The central ray of the x-ray beam is then directed perpendicularly at this bisecting line. This will project the proper linear dimensions of the tooth onto the film without elongation or foreshortening.

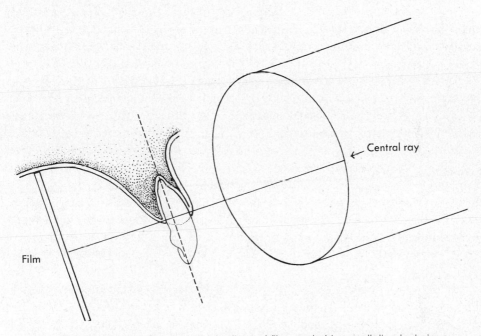

Film

Central ray

Fig. 1-29. Relationship of central ray, tooth, and film packet in paralleling technique.

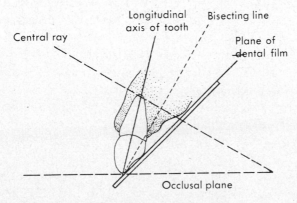

Central ray

Longitudinal axis of tooth

Bisecting line

Plane of dental film

Occlusal plane

Fig. 1-30. Relationship of central ray, tooth, and film packet in bisecting-angle technique.

FILM

Dental intraoral film packets come in three basic sizes (Fig. 1-31): child size, #0, adult size, #2, and narrow anterior film, #1. There are also occlusal film packets, #4, and preformed long bite-wing films, #3, available.

All the film packets must be light-tight and resistant to saliva seepage. These packets must have some degree of flexibility and should be easy to open in the darkroom.

The dental x-ray film packet has an outer plasticlike wrapper. Inside the wrapper is found the x-ray film, covered by black paper, and a lead-foil backing. The lead backing is placed on the side of the film away from the x-ray tube to absorb any unused radiation and prevent backscattering secondary radiation from fogging the film (Fig. 1-32).

A film packet may contain one or two pieces of film. The so-called double film packet requires slightly more exposure time than the single film packet.

X-ray film is composed of a clear cellulose acetate film base coated with a silver halide emulsion and covered by gelatin. The film base is coated on both sides and thus is called a double emulsion. Clinically, this means that a radiograph can be correctly viewed from either side. Previously, with single emulsion film the film had to be viewed from the side with the emulsion on it. The film also has a button or dot on it. This is a small convex-concave area that helps one to orient the developed film in mounting (see Chapter 8).

The silver halide emulsion is usually silver bromide crystals, bromides being of the halide family.

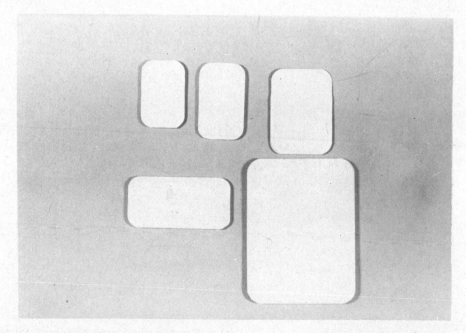

Fig. 1-31. Intraoral film packet sizes, child (#0); narrow anterior (#1); adult size (#2); preformed bite-wing (#3); and occlusal (#4).

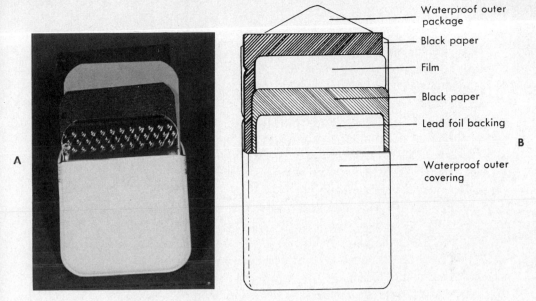

Waterproof outer package

Black paper

Film

Black paper

Lead foil backing

Waterproof outer covering

B

A

Fig. 1-32. A, Back of an opened dental film packet. **B,** Diagram of A.

Film sensitivity

The size of the silver bromide crystals determines the film speed, or film sensitivity. Film sensitivity determines how much radiation for what period of time (mAs) will be necessary to produce an image on the film. Films that are more sensitive require less mAs and are said to have greater film speed; these are the fast films. Films that require more mAs are less sensitive to radiation and are called slower films. The size of the silver bromide crystals determines the film speed: the larger the crystals, the faster the film.

Different film manufacturers will give different brand names to their various film speed types. There is no slow-speed film being made today. At 65 kVp and 10 mA, slow film would need an average exposure time of about 3 seconds per film. Under the same conditions the intermediate-speed film would need about 1½ seconds and the fast film about 3/10-second exposure per film. One manufacturer's "Ultraspeed" (Eastman Kodak Co.) may be equal to another's "lightning" or "very fast" film speed. It is obvious that some standards are necessary. Film speed is designated into groups by the American National Standards Institute (ANSI) using the letters A through F, A being the slowest film and F the fastest. To get comparable film sensitivities when changing from one manufacturer to another, one should consult the ANSI speed group ratings found on the package and not be misled by descriptive names.

The American Dental Association currently recommends the use of ANSI Group D films or faster.[2] Many health codes have prohibited the use of any dental film slower than ANSI Group D, and very few major manufacturers have continued to make intraoral dental film slower than Group D. Recently, the Eastman Kodak Company introduced "Ektaspeed" film, which is ANSI Group E. This new film is twice as fast, requiring half the exposure time of Group D films.

39

Film definition and detail

The definition or detail on a film is also dependent on the size of the silver bromide crystals. The larger crystals, although they allow for reduced exposure time, give poorer definition when compared with the smaller, slower crystals.

The dilemma is whether to reduce the amount of radiation the patient receives by using fast films with large crystals, thereby sacrificing definition, or to increase exposure time by using small crystals to give better definition and thereby increase radiation exposure. This is largely a theoretical dilemma, because the human eye, which must view the finished radiograph, cannot easily distinguish between the definition on intermediate-speed films and that on fast films.

Film fog

An x-ray film is fogged when the whole or part of the radiograph is darkened by sources other than the radiation of the primary beam to which the film was exposed. Fogging degrades the diagnostic image. The following are several sources of fogging:

1. Chemical fog results from an imbalance or exhaustion of processing solutions (see Chapter 7).
2. Light fog results from unintentional exposure of light to which the film emulsion is sensitive, either before or during processing (see Chapter 7).
3. Radiation fog results from radiation striking the film from sources other than the intentional exposure of the primary beam. Examples of this would be scatter from the patient or unprotected storage of films before or after exposure.

XERORADIOGRAPHY

Xeroradiography is an imaging system, as is conventional dental film, that has been used in medical radiology for some time. The system uses the xerographic copying process to record images produced by x-rays from a standard dental x-ray machine. The system does not replace the conventional x-ray unit. It replaces film as the imaging system. Instead of conventional film, a photoreceptor plate covered with a uniform charge is used as the image receptor. The charged plate is held in a light-tight cassette which is the size of either #0 or #2 film. The cassette is covered with a plastic bag and is exposed intra-orally in the routine manner by a dental x-ray machine. The x-rays dissipate the charge on the photoreceptor plate in a pattern that corresponds to the absorption of the x-rays by the object being radiographed. A latent electrostatic image is thus formed.

The exposed receptor plate is then placed back into the processing machine and the latent image is transformed into a real image on opaque paper that can be viewed directly or by reflected light on a viewbox. This is done by the use of a specifically charged pigmented powder. This copying process takes 20 seconds. After the photoreceptor plate is sterilized, reconditioned, and recharged, it is ready to be used again. Gratt and White using the xeroradiographic system have reported superior image quality and a radiation dose one third those of conventional films.[3] (Figs. 1-33 and 1-34).

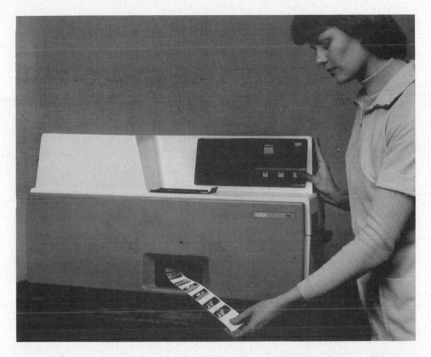

Fig. 1-33. The Xerox 110 Dental Diagnostic Imaging System. (Courtesy Xerox Medical Systems, Pasadena, Calif.)

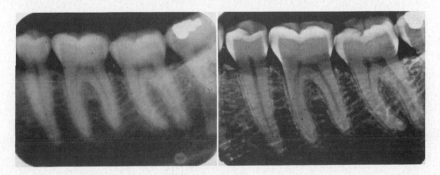

Fig. 1-34. Conventional dental radiograph *(left)* and xeroradiograph *(right)* of same area. (Courtesy Xerox Medical Systems, Pasadena, Calif.)

STUDY QUESTIONS

1. What are radiations? List the important properties of x-rays and explain how they apply to clinical dentistry.
2. Explain the similarities and differences between x-rays and visible light.
3. Make a drawing of the dental x-ray tube and its component parts. List the functions of each part.
4. Explain the difference between filtration and collimation of the x-ray beam. What are the requirements of each?
5. What is rectangular collimation? Why is it important?
6. Explain the difference between kilovoltage and milliamperage and what they control in the dental x-ray machine.
7. Explain the following terms and sketch examples of each: object-film distance; focal-film distance; divergent and parallel rays of the x-ray beam.
8. What factors determine the density and contrast of the finished radiograph?
9. What is the ideal relationship for intraoral radiography between the x-ray tube, tooth, and film packet? Can this be achieved? Why or why not?
10. What is the importance of target (focal) area size?
11. What is ionization? Describe how x-rays produce ionization.
12. Does the patient receive greater exposure to radiation with the longer exposure in the 16-inch FFD when compared with a comparable radiograph using an 8-inch FFD?
13. What determines film speed? What film speed should be used?
14. What is the purpose of the lead foil in the film packet?
15. What is film fog and what are its causes?

REFERENCES

1. Performance standards for electronic products: diagnostic x-ray systems and their major components, Fed. Register **37**:16461, 1972.
2. American Dental Association, Council on Dental Materials, Instruments, and Equipment: Recommendations in radiographic practices, 1981, J. Am. Dent. Assoc. **103**:103, July 1981.
3. Gratt, B.M., and others: Imaging properties of intraoral dental xeroradiography, J. Am. Dent. Assoc. **99**:805, November 1979.

chapter 2 Radiation protection

Much has been written, not only in scientific journals but also in the lay press, about the effects of ionizing radiation, both man-made and naturally occurring, on human beings and the environment. This growing concern about the biologic effects of ionizing radiation is not limited to the scientific community but is evident in the public sector and at all levels of government. Events such as the nuclear accident at Three Mile Island, Pennsylvania, have heightened public awareness to the dangers of low-level radiation. Demands are being put on government for more stringent control over all types of ionizing radiation, including dental use.

The Consumer Patient Radiation Health and Safety Act of 1981 is such a response. In this bill the United States Congress has mandated that the Department of Health and Human Services develop standards for accreditation and certification of "persons who administer radiologic procedures" other than a practitioner. The targeted groups of this new federal legislation include dental assistants and hygienists.

Information about ionizing radiation that reaches the public from the media can be misleading and confusing. Patient reaction can vary from questioning the need for dental radiographs to outright refusal. The dental auxiliary must face this patient reaction and, with the support of the dentist, be able to explain to the patient the biologic effects of dental x-ray exposure and the diagnostic benefits that will be derived.

Ionizing radiation does produce biologic changes in living tissue and patients should not be misled into believing that dental x-rays have no effect on human cells. The old reply to patient queries regarding radiation safety that claimed that, "Dental x-rays are safe because the dosage is so small it doesn't matter," will not longer satisfy the informed public.

The question no longer is if there is a risk from dental x-rays, but how much of a risk there is. In determining if radiographs should be used, the dental auxiliary, as well as the dentist, must weigh the potential harm of dental x-rays against the benefit the diagnostic information will yield. In dental radiography performed under optimum conditions and when indicated, the diagnostic benefits far outweigh the potential risks.

Our objective for the patient is to use the least possible amount of radiation to obtain the greatest diagnostic yield. For the dental auxiliary, as well as the dentist, our objective is to achieve occupational radiation exposure as close to zero as possible. To achieve these objectives the dental auxiliary must fully understand the subjects of radiation biology and protection. Explanations to patients will then be meaningful, and the assistant or hygienist will feel at ease working with radiation.

BIOLOGIC EFFECTS OF RADIATION

When a dental radiograph is taken, not all the x-rays reach the film and some even penetrate beyond it. Some of the x-ray energy of the primary beam is dissipated by the skin, bones, teeth, and other body tissues that lie in its path. Tissues that do not lie in the path of the primary beam dissipate the energy of the secondary radiation that comes from the patient. It is the differential absorption of the x-ray photons by the hard tissues, teeth, and bone that enables us to distinguish various structures on the finished radiograph. What is the effect of this x-ray energy absorption on the various tissues, and how is it manifested?

The human body, like all living organisms, functions through the existence of ions in its organs, tissues, and cells. These ions are electrically charged particles that originate in the water, salts, proteins, carbohydrates, and fats, which are the principal ingredients of our bodies. The ions affect the many complex functions that maintain the health of the body and that return it to health after illness. Ions are ever present in a finely balanced state, or equilibrium, so that precise control over the reactions concerned with body function can be maintained. If an overabundance of ions occurs, the surplus must be removed immediately if health is to be maintained; illness will also occur if an insufficient number of necessary ions is available for essential functioning. Special ions maintain the proper body environment for such things as respiration, muscular activity, speech, and digestion. X-ray exposure, depending on the amount, can upset this delicately balanced state.

One of the characteristics of x-rays is the ability to cause ionization, or the production of ions, when they interact with matter. In the case of interaction with or penetration of the human body, extra ions become available. These extra ions can upset the fine ionic balance that exists. If the amount of radiation exposure is large, there will be a great ionic upset and the body will react by showing signs of injury or illness. It is important to understand that x-rays are ionizing radiations and, as such, have the potential to affect the health of the human body.

BASIC CONCEPTS

Exposure and dose

Although the terms are often interchanged, there is a very definite distinction between radiation exposure and dose. Exposure is the measure of ionization in the air produced by x-ray or gamma radiation; it is the quantity of radiation in an area to which the patient is exposed. The radiation dose is the amount of energy absorbed per unit mass of tissue at a particular site. In dentistry, the patient is exposed to a certain amount of radiation, some of which is absorbed by tissue in different parts of the body; this is the dose to the area.

Measurement of radiation—roentgen, rad, rem

Before we can talk logically about the potential effects of dental radiation we must have some means of measuring the radiation quantitatively. The settings on the control panel of the dental x-ray machine are not measurements of the x-ray energy (ionizing radiation) produced; the kilovoltage and milliamperage are indications of the quality and quantity of the electric energy put into the x-ray machine, and the timer provides a reading of how long the ionizing radiation will be produced. The unit most commonly used to measure the amount of energy, or ionizing radiation, being produced by the x-ray machine is called the *roentgen* and is abbreviated as R. A *milliroentgen* is $1/1000$ of a roentgen; because the exposure dosages in dental radiology are small, they are often expressed in milliroentgens, or mR (1000 mR = 1 R).

The roentgen is a measurement of ionization in air. It is defined as the unit of exposure dose that produces one electrostatic charge in 1 cc of air. The roentgen is our measuring standard for radiation. Just as we have to know what an inch is before we can compare lengths, we have a standard, the roentgen, to measure radiation. Just as there are rulers and scales, there are roentgen meters. A roentgen meter can be placed in front of a dental x-ray machine PID and indicate how many roentgens are being produced per second (Fig. 2-1). This is called the exposure rate or output of the machine. Since it is a measurement of ionization in air, it is measured in roentgens per second. A well-calibrated dental x-ray machine will have an output in the range of 0.7 to 1 R per second. If a patient had a radiograph taken with such a machine and the exposure time were 1 second, the facial exposure of the patient would be 0.7 R (0.7 R/sec × 1 sec = 0.7 R). Radiation can also be expressed in the amount of energy absorbed by the tissue. The unit of absorbed dose is the *rad* (radiation absorbed dose). The rad is defined as 100 ergs of energy per gram of absorber. In dental x-rays 1 roentgen is approximately equal to 1 rad of absorbed dose.

The *rem* is an acronym for roentgen equivalent man. It is the dose of radiation that will produce the same biologic effects in humans as are produced by the absorption of

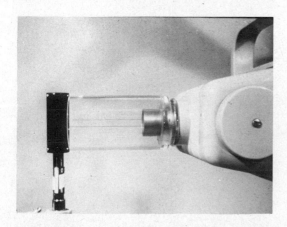

Fig. 2-1. Roentgen meter measuring the output of dental x-ray machine.

1 R of x radiation. The rem is the product of the absorbed dose in rads and certain qualifying factors (rem = rad × QF). The rem takes into consideration that different types of radiations will have different effects on human tissue. It is the unit used to measure the dose equivalent or relative biologic effectiveness (RBE). For example, the qualifying factor for diagnostic x-rays, both medical and dental, is one, so for dental purposes the rem equals the rad. For radiation such as neutron radiation (for example, the radiation produced by a neutron bomb) the qualifying factor would be twenty, and thus much more damaging to human tissue.

In discussions of dental radiation the roentgen, rad, and rem, although they have different meanings, can be considered equal.

Other units of radiation measurement to be familiar with include the *curie, gray, sievert,* and *becquerel.* The curie measures the radioactivity produced by the disintegration of unstable elements; it is the number of nuclear disintegrations per second, not the amount of radiation emitted. The becquerel is to be placed into general use by 1985 to replace the curie. Also to be placed into use by 1985 are the gray and the sievert. The gray will become the unit of absorbed dose and replace the rad (1 Gy = 100 rads). The sievert will become the unit of dose equivalent and replace the rem.

These terms, like the roentgen, are the names of pioneers in the field of radiation.

Dose response curve

The dose response curve is an important concept because it illustrates the two possible biologic responses to a harmful agent such as ionizing radiation. Fig. 2-2, *A,* is a threshold curve indicating that below a certain level (the threshold) there is no response to the agent. If this concept is applied to dental radiation, there would be a level below which radiographs would be "perfectly safe" since there would be no biologic response below that level. This is not thought to be the case for ionizing radiation. As shown in Fig. 2-2, *B,* the consensus is that the response to ionizing radiation is a linear, nonthreshold relationship.[1] This means that any dose of radiation, regardless of how small, will produce some degree of biologic response. Therefore, dental x-rays do produce biologic changes in the tissues of the patients who receive them.

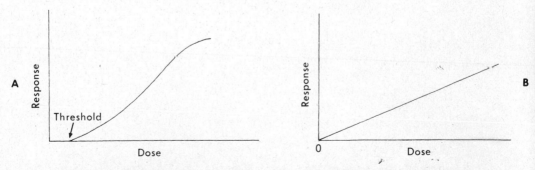

Fig. 2-2. Dose response curve. **A,** Threshold curve. **B,** Nonthreshold linear type.

Localized radiation and total body exposure (Fig. 2-3)

It is important to differentiate between localized radiation and total body exposure. When a dental radiograph is taken, the patient's face is exposed to an x-ray beam that is 2¾ inches in diameter (with circular collimation). This is a localized exposure to that area of the body. A rad of radiation to the localized area means that each gram of body tissue in that area absorbs 1 rad of radiation. A rad of total body radiation means that each gram of tissue in the entire body absorbs 1 rad of radiation. In dentistry the machine delivers a localized exposure that results in a total body exposure much less than the facial exposure. In fact, the total body exposure from a dental radiograph is approximately ¹/₁₀,₀₀₀ of the facial exposure.

When discussions of dental x-ray dosages appear in magazine articles, or if patients quote such articles, it is important to determine if localized exposure or total body exposure is being discussed. For instance, what is the facial exposure of radiation to the patient from a full-mouth survey of radiographs? An average full-mouth survey at 65 kVp, 10 mA, using ANSI Group D film, will produce a skin exposure to the patient's face of approximately 3 to 5 R. This is not the total body exposure but a localized exposure. The total body exposure could be calculated by dividing the localized dose, 3 R, by 10,000.

The most common misuse of data of this kind occurs when referring to the recommendation of the National Bureau of Standards that the total body dose for people working with ionizing radiation should not exceed 5 R in any 1 year. The misstatement then is, "You are allowed 5 R per year, and when your dentist x-rays your entire mouth he exposes you to 3 R of radiation." The mistake here is equating the total body dose to the localized dose in addition to using an occupational dose for a patient dose. The truer figure to compare the dental facial dose with the 5 R would be 0.0003 R.

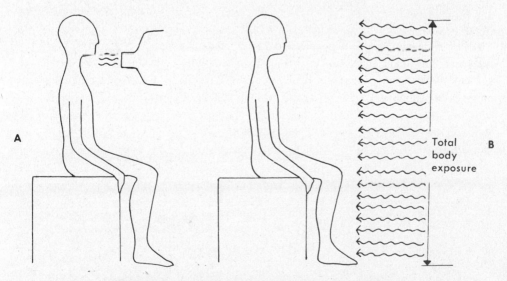

Fig. 2-3. A, Localized exposure. **B,** Total body exposure.

Acute and chronic effects

The short-term (acute) effects of radiation result from high doses of whole body radiation, usually over 100 rads. The clinical effect of the exposure, which may vary from mild and transient illness to death, may occur minutes, hours, or weeks after the acute exposure. The median lethal dose for humans is estimated to be 450 rads. It is obvious that in dentistry we are not concerned with acute radiation doses.

Long-term (chronic) effects of radiation may be seen years after the original exposures. There may be cumulative effects of acute and/or chronic exposures to the somatic cells over the patient's lifetime, as well as genetic effects on future generations.

Somatic and genetic effects

All the cells in the body, with the exception of the reproductive cells (sperm and ova), are included in the grouping of somatic tissue. Changes in these cells are not passed on to succeeding generations of the species. For example, a cancerous skin condition will not be passed on to an offspring. Somatic tissue can be affected by radiation and some cells may die, be altered, or even recover, but none of these effects will be seen in the somatic tissue of the progeny.

Changes in genetic cells are passed on to succeeding generations and are referred to as genetic mutations. There are many other agents besides ionizing radiation that have been found to be mutanogenic, including a variety of chemicals, certain drugs, and elevated body temperatures. Background radiation also accounts for a portion of naturally occurring mutations. Some of the mutations that have been manifested have been positive and have aided in the so-called evolution of the species. A mutation may be recessive and carried in the progeny for many generations before becoming clinically evident.

With the increase in low-level man-made radiation in recent years, the original concern dealt mainly with the possible genetic effects on succeeding generations. Recently the concern has turned toward somatic tissue and the blood-forming organs in particular; leukemia induction is now the major risk of chronic low-level radiation.

The National Academy of Sciences has recommended that "the average exposure of the populations' reproductive cells to radiation above natural background levels should be limited to ten roentgens from conception to age thirty."[2] The gonadal exposure from a dental full-mouth survey has been reported in the range of .0004 to .07 R, before the introduction of Group E film, thus putting dental gonadal exposure within acceptable limits.[3] It is estimated that the gonadal dose in dental radiography is about $1/10,000$ the facial dose. The genetic risk for the dental patient, exposed under proper conditions, would appear rather small.

Direct and indirect effects

The effects of ionizing radiation on tissue may be direct, as when the ionizing radiation alters or destroys cells that lie in the direct path of the radiation beam. The effects may also be indirect, as when the impaired function of the radiated tissue adversely influences other tissues in the body. An example of an indirect effect would be the production of a chemically changed hormone that could not properly regulate tissue elsewhere in the body.

Latent period and cell recovery

The latent period is the time that elapses between the exposure to ionizing radiation and the appearance of clinical symptoms. This time may vary from hours to years, depending on the magnitude of the exposure and the tissues involved. Not all radiation-induced changes in tissue cells are permanent. Depending on the time interval, the dose, and the sensitivity of the affected cells to radiation, the cells repair processes may be sufficient to affect recovery from the radiation.

Dose rate

The *dose rate,* the rate at which exposure to ionizing radiation occurs and absorption takes place, is a very important factor in determining what the effects will be. Since there is cell recovery from radiation, a specific dose will produce less damage if it is fractionated over a period of time. In dentistry, the time interval between exposures, excluding retakes and working films, is usually months or years, further minimizing the effects.

Tissue sensitivity

There is a wide variation among tissues in their sensitivity to ionizing radiation and thus the amount of radiation required to produce damage. The same dose of radiation will have a different degree of effect on different types of cells in the same organism. Young, rapidly dividing, nondifferentiated cells, such as those found in the abdomen of the pregnant dental patient, are more radiosensitive than older cells. Grouping tissues and organs in descending order of sensitivity to radiation, we have the following:
1. Reproductive cells and blood-forming tissue
2. Glandular tissue, young bone, and alimentary epithelium
3. Skin and muscle tissue
4. Nerve tissue and adult bone

Certain organs and tissues have been designated as ''critical'' because of their potential harmful effect upon the patient. The critical organs or tissues are the skin, thyroid, eye, and hematopoietic and genetic tissue.

BACKGROUND RADIATION

Background radiation is a form of ionizing radiation, both naturally occurring and man-made, present in the environment. This naturally occurring radiation has always been present on earth, but the man-made component has been increasing as a result of fallout from nuclear testing and radioactive wastes from industry. Before we discuss the radiation exposure delivered by the dental machine, it would be helpful to know the level of background radiation and its sources, so that dental radiation exposure can be put in its proper perspective.

The average background radiation for the world's population is thought to be 100 mR per year. That is, we are all exposed to 100 mR of total body radiation just by being on earth. The following are the four major sources of this radiation:

1. Cosmic rays. Cosmic rays are rays from the sun. People who live at higher altitudes are affected more than those who live at sea level. These rays account for a range of 28 mR per year at sea level to 45 mR per year at an altitude of 5000 feet.
2. External radiation. External radiation comes from radioactive materials found naturally in the earth that are incorporated into building materials that give off gamma rays. It accounts for a range of 40 to 60 mR per year.
3. Internal radiation. Certain radioactive materials are ingested. For example, potassium 40, a radioactive isotope of potassium, which is an essential component of a normal diet, represents 0.01% of all potassium ingested. Internal radiation accounts for about 20 mR per year of background radiation.
4. Fallout. Fallout from nuclear explosives accounts for about 2 to 5 mR per year exposure to the population. It is hoped that this component of background radiation can be kept to an absolute minimum.

DENTAL RADIATION EXPOSURE

Primary and secondary radiation

Primary radiation is the energy contained by the x-rays that come from the target of the x-ray tube. The primary radiation is collimated by the lead diaphragm and filtered of its softer wavelengths by aluminum filters. It is then referred to as the useful beam. All other radiation can be considered secondary radiation. *Secondary radiation* is defined as radiation that comes from any matter being struck by primary radiation. The scattered radiation that results from the interaction of the useful beam and the patient's face is a form of secondary radiation (Fig. 2-4). Secondary radiation, besides being harmful to both patient and operator, will degrade the diagnostic image of the film; the scattered rays will produce film fog on the radiograph. Two of the main thrusts of radiation protection are (1) to limit the size of the beam of primary radiation and (2) to decrease the patient's exposure to secondary radiation. The dentist and dental auxiliary should never be in the path of the useful beam of primary radiation and should be protected from exposure to secondary radiation.

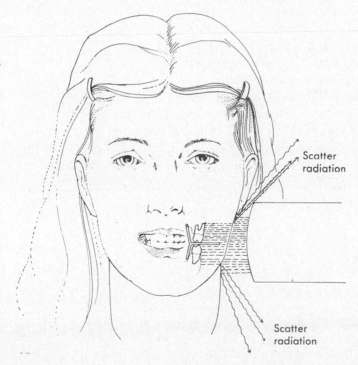

Scatter radiation

Scatter radiation

Fig. 2-4. Production of scatter radiation of primary beam by interaction with patient's face.

PATIENT DOSAGE

Our aim, in the use of dental x-rays, is always to use the least amount of radiation to satisfy the patient's diagnostic needs; that is, minimize the exposure while maximizing the diagnostic yield. To treat a patient without current and valid radiographs is doing a disservice to the patient and leaves the dentist unprotected against possible malpractice suits. In considering patient dosage, we should follow the ALARA principle—as low as reasonably achievable. The dose to the patient should be reduced as much as possible without excessive cost or inconvenience; any dose that can be avoided without undue consequences should be avoided.

Effects

Since the dental x-ray exposure to the patient is relatively low there are no acute (short-term) effects. The concern for our patients is with the chronic (long-term) effects of all low-level exposures, of which dental x-rays are just one component. From a public health viewpoint there is much greater concern for large populations that receive low-level chronic exposures than for a few individuals that may receive acute exposures.

How do we evaluate these effects of ionizing radiation and the weight of the dental component? There is no specific disease that can be attributed solely to the long-term effects of ionizing radiation. Leukemia, for example, is not caused by x-ray exposure alone but is probably the result of the interaction of several factors. Animal experimentation has been done but direct extrapolation of the results of human populations is not always reliable. Data gained from acute exposures of humans, as in victims of Hiroshima or industrial accidents, that are then extrapolated downward to low doses, also have their limitations. Furthermore, the incidence of the diseases we are concerned with is low, so in order to relate an increased incidence with population exposure to ionizing radiations it is necessary to study large populations. Dental auxiliaries and dentists, because of their involvement with low-level ionizing radiation, should be aware of the consequences of chronic exposure for their patients. In this manner, they are better equipped to make the essential ''risk vs benefit'' decision before making x-ray exposures.

The following examples of specific tissue exposures from dental x-ray exposure and the critical levels of these tissues enable us to say that the benefits derived from dental x-ray exposure, when used judiciously under proper conditions, far outweigh any possible risk.

Skin. Erythema (reddening of the skin) is not a major concern in dental radiography. There has never been a case of erythema reported as a result of exposure to dental radiation.[3] The threshold erythema dose (TED), the amount of radiation needed to produce an erythema or reddening of the most sensitive individual, is 250 R in a 14-day period. Assuming an exposure rate of 0.7 R/sec from a dental x-ray machine, using ANSI Group D film, more than 250 dental exposures in a 14-day period would be necessary to produce an erythema in the most sensitive patient. This would be an example of an acute effect.

Eyes. Exposure to ionizing radiation in high doses can induce cataract formation. The required dose to produce this change has been reported in the range of 200 to 2000 rads,[3] while the mean corneal surface dose for a full-mouth series is about 0.188 rad.[4] The important fact is that there is a dose to the eye during dental radiography, and although alone it may not be significant, it must be considered part of the patient's total exposure.

Hair. Loss of hair, alopecia, has never been reported as a result of exposure to radiation from dental exposures.

Thyroid. The thyroid gland, which is particularly radiosensitive, may lie in the beam of primary radiation in some dental views. Malignant changes have been reported in the thyroid glands in a group of patients who received x-ray therapy for tinea capitis (ringworm of the scalp). The dose to the thyroid in these patients was estimated to be 6 rads. Presently, the thyroid exposure for a full-mouth series is about 25 mR, or about 0.3% of the exposure in the tinea capitis studies.[5] The dose to this radiosensitive tissue should be kept to an absolute minimum, especially in children. This can be accomplished by the use of a lead thryoid collar.

Blood. Although the blood-forming organs are extremely radiosensitive, it has been demonstrated that there are no acute hematologic changes after dental x-ray examination.[6] This refutes the earlier report that claimed significant blood changes after dental x-rays.[7]

With regard to the long-term effects of radiation, it is thought that the greatest somatic hazard to the population from dental x-rays is leukemia induction.[8] However, the hazard is probably very low and with judicious use and proper technique, the potential risk does not outweigh the diagnostic benefit derived.

Carcinogenic effect. There is little doubt that ionizing radiation at certain dose levels has a carcinogenic action on organs and tissues. There is ample evidence from both laboratory and epidemiologic studies of irradiated subjects to support this conclusion.[1] Dental exposures alone do not cause cancer but do add to the patient's overall radiation burden.

Pregnancy. As was previously mentioned, the nondifferentiated, rapidly dividing fetal cells are extremely radiosensitive and hence the problem of the pregnant patient. The second through the sixth weeks of gestation have been called the most critical in regard to the production of congenital anomalies. This is also the period of the unsuspected pregnancy, in which neither the patient nor the dentist may take the radiographic precautions associated with pregnancy. These factors, coupled with the fact that the head of the x-ray machine is close to the patient's abdomen during many projections, has caused great concern.

53

Patients of childbearing age should always be asked if they are pregnant or could *possibly* be pregnant. If the patient is pregnant, only radiographs deemed essential to treatment that cannot be postponed until after the pregnancy should be taken. The minimum number of exposures should be used and the patient, like all other patients, should be draped with a lead apron. There are modifying factors in the risk vs benefit concept that tip the scale to the risk side and necessitate a modified approach.

Gonads (sperm cells and ova). The reproductive cells, sperm in the male and ova in the female, are very radiosensitive. Sterilization from an acute exposure from the dental x-ray beam is an impossibility; 400 R is needed in the male and 625 R in the female to cause sterility.

PATIENT PROTECTION

The patient must be adequately protected to achieve the goals of the risk vs benefit concept for the use of ionizing radiation. The patient is protected from overexposure to primary radiation and the effects of secondary radiation. Through the use of safe, well-calibrated equipment, good chairside and darkroom technique, and sound professional judgment, these goals can be met.

Equipment

The term *head leakage* refers to radiation that escapes through the protective shielding of the x-ray tube head. The only radiation that should leave the tube head is the primary beam. Radiation leakage exposes the patient unnecessarily and should not occur in a properly functioning x-ray unit. Leakage is a violation of the Federal Performance Standards and local radiation codes.[9]

Filtration and collimation

Because of the enactment of certain statutes filtration and collimation are no longer major concerns in patient protection. Dental x-ray machines manufactured and installed after August 1, 1974, must have filtration and collimation that conforms to the Federal Performance Standards (see Chapter 1).[9] Those units manufactured and installed before 1974 are subject to the same requirements under state and local health codes.

The purpose of filtration is to remove the soft, nonpenetrating x-ray photons from the x-ray beam. These photons would either be absorbed by the overlying tissue or give rise to secondary radiation that would not benefit the patient or the quality of the image. Collimation limits the size of the area exposed by the primary beam and the amount of scatter produced. Rectangular collimation can be achieved by using either a lead-lined open-ended rectangular PID (see Fig. 1-24) or a metallic film-holding shield with a rectangular opening (Fig. 2-5). This type of collimation is highly recommended for increased patient protection.

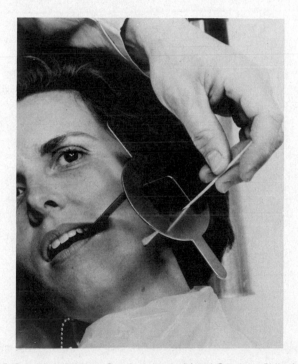

Fig. 2-5. Precision device. (Courtesy Isaac Masel Co., Inc., Philadelphia.)

Timing device

The use of more sensitive x-ray film with extremely short exposure times makes the use of electronic timers imperative. All new x-ray machines come equipped in this manner.

The mechanical timers existing on older machines are inaccurate at short exposures and are usually calibrated down to ¼ second. It is impossible to use a mechanical timer with Group D and E film and make accurate exposures. Mechanical timers should be replaced by the electronic type.

Position indicating devices

Open-ended lead-lined cylinders or rectangles are the PID of choice (Fig. 2-6). The use of closed and pointed cones is contraindicated (see Chapter 1). These cones increase the scattered radiation to the patient because of the interaction of the primary beam with the plastic cone (see Fig. 1-12).

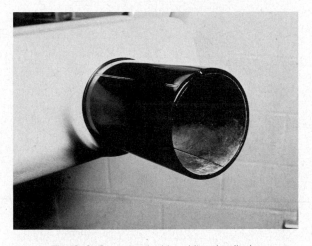

Fig. 2-6. Open-ended lead-lined cylinder.

Film

Decreasing the exposure time by the use of a more sensitive receptor (film) is probably the single most important factor in reducing exposure to the patient. The American Dental Association, through its Council on Dental Materials, Instruments and Equipment, has recommended that for periapical and bite-wing radiography, "Only film of ANSI Speed Group D rating or faster should be used."[10]

Faster or Group E film is now available and being marketed by the Eastman Kodak Company under the trade name "Ektaspeed." The Group E film is twice as fast as the Group D film and thus reduces the patient exposure by one half.[11] This is a significant step forward in patient protection and all dental auxiliaries and dentists should be using the faster film. Its use requires an electronic timer and strict adherence to time-temperature processing because the film has very little leeway for error. The possible slight lowering of contrast and loss of detail, which is not apparent without magnification, are far outweighed by the 50% reduction in patient exposure.

Lead aprons (Fig. 2-7)

All patients should be draped with a lead apron during dental x-ray exposures. This rule should be adhered to regardless of the patient's age or the number of films being exposed. The apron should cover the patient from the thyroid to the gonadal area. The aprons available are usually the equivalent of 0.25 mm lead, relatively light and flexible, and not uncomfortable for the patient. There is no valid reason not to use a lead apron for every exposure. Many states have enacted legislation that makes this procedure mandatory.

Lead aprons should not be folded when not in use. Folding will eventually crack the lead and allow leakage.

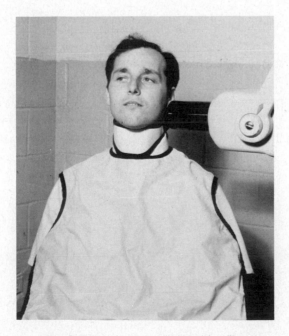

Fig. 2-7. Lead apron with thyroid collar.

Technique

Retakes. One of the major sources of unnecessary exposure to radiation in the dental office is the retaking of films due to poor technique in either the taking or processing of films. Every retake represents an unnecessary doubling of radiation exposure to the patient for that film. It is the obligation of both the dental auxiliary and the dentist to perfect their intraoral technique so that retakes will be unnecessary.

Exposure. Films should be exposed properly. A technique that employs overexposure with underdevelopment subjects the patient to unnecessary radiation. If exposed films come out too dark upon time-temperature processing, the exposure time, not the developing time, should be reduced. An overexposure and a shortened processing time used to expedite patient treatment is unconscionable in relation to good patient radiation hygiene.

Focal-film distance. Increased FFDs, up to 16 inches, are recommended with the paralleling technique to compensate for the magnification of the image caused by the increased object-film distance (see Chapter 1). Another important advantage of an increased FFD is that there is less total body area in the path of the primary beam at 16 inches than at 8 inches. As the distance increases from 8 to 16 inches (Fig. 2-8), the x-ray beam becomes less divergent and there is less total body area irradiated by the primary beam after it penetrates the skin. The shorter FFD, with a more divergent beam, irradiates a far greater volume of tissue. The diameter of the primary beam is still 2¾ inches at the skin in both cases. The difference is in the beam divergence after the skin entry and film exposure.

Darkroom. Every effort should be made to establish darkroom procedures that will produce films with the maximum diagnostic yield. As previously mentioned, underdevelopment should not compensate for overexposure. There is no excuse for darkroom errors that cause retaking of films.

Viewing finished radiographs

In order to get the maximum diagnostic yield for the radiation expended, the manner in which radiographs are viewed for interpretation is extremely important. The only proper way to view a radiograph is in front of an illuminator (viewbox), preferably with a variable light source. Using sunlight in front of a window or the lamp on the dental unit is unsatisfactory. The film mount used for the full-mouth survey should cover the entire illuminator and empty windows in the mount should be covered with an opaque material. This will prevent light that escapes around the periphery or through the mount from distracting the viewer. Ideally, the radiographs should be viewed in a darkened room to avoid excessive reflection.

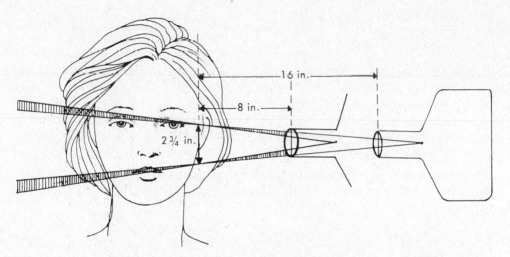

Fig. 2-8. Focal-film distance and tissue volume exposed. Shaded areas represent tissue that is exposed at 8-inch FFD but not in the beam at 16-inch FFD because of the more parallel and less divergent x-rays.

PROFESSIONAL JUDGMENT

The following decisions should be made by the dentist following the risk vs benefit concept and the needs of the individual patient:
1. What type of radiograph should be taken?
2. When should radiographs be taken?
3. How many radiographs should be taken?

The selection criteria are based on professional judgment. There are no such things as "routine dental radiographs." Radiographic needs are not determined by the calendar but rather by evaluating the overall health needs of a patient after a clinical examination and history. This is true for new patients, emergencies, and recall visits.

Radiation history

Specific questions regarding the patient's prior exposures should be part of every history. This should include medical, dental, and therapeutic exposures. Questions of this type may help determine if there have been dental x-rays taken recently that might be available and still diagnostically valid. Patients may not volunteer such information on their own, thinking it is not important.

Selection criteria

Recently specific criteria have been offered regarding the frequency and number of radiographs taken,[12,13] but the final decision rests with the individual dentist and is determined by professional judgment.

All new patients should have a recent full-mouth survey on file before treatment is instituted. They may have been taken by the present dentist or duplicates of those taken by a previous dentist. The full-mouth survey is essential for case planning, baseline data for future reference, and medical-legal reasons.

Recall radiographs should not be taken on all patients as a matter of routine. Very few, if any, patients need radiographs at 6-month intervals. Caries susceptibility should be considered when determining the time frame for recall radiographs. The diagnostic radiographic needs of a decay-prone teenager are quite different from a middle-aged periodontal recall patient whose last filling was placed 20 years earlier.

Postoperative radiographs are indicated only when they have diagnostic value, for example, confirming the retrieval of a root tip in surgery. The use of radiographs to check the fit, contact, contour, and seating of restorations should be discouraged. This is best done with a mirror, explorer, and floss, thus saving the patient the radiation exposure.

Working films in endodontics, surgery, and restorative post and pin preparations may be necessary for proper treatment, but every effort should be made to keep the number of exposures to a minimum.

Administrative radiographs, those taken to verify treatment for compensation by insurance companies or other third-party carriers, should never be taken for that purpose alone. Many states have legislation that prohibits their use and the Food and Drug Administration has recommended that insurance carriers, etc. refrain from requiring administrative radiographs.[14]

OPERATOR DOSAGE AND PROTECTION

Of the two concerns in radiation protection, operator and patient, the operator is much easier to deal with. The sources of potential exposure to the dental auxiliary are the primary beam, head leakage from the tube, and secondary radiation originating from the patient, x-ray machine, or objects in the operatory. Through the use of careful technique, in a well-designed, well-equipped, and well-monitored office, the occupational dose to dental auxiliaries and dentists can be kept to a minimum.

Maximum permissible dose

At present, the maximum permissible dose (MPD) of whole body radiation for persons occupationally concerned with ionizing radiation, such as the dental auxiliary and dentist, is 5 rem per year or 100 millirem per week. In addition, the operator should not receive more than 3 rem in any 13 week period. Dental personnel also should not exceed an accumluated lifetime dose of $(N - 18) \times 5$ rem. In this formula, N is the operator's age.

Although 5 rem is the stated MPD, dental auxiliaries and dentists should strive for an occupational dose of zero. It is not difficult to achieve this in an office where there is an awareness of radiation hygiene. One should not fear working with x-rays but should be knowledgeable about their use and abuse.

Radiation monitoring

How can dental auxiliaries and dentists know the amount of occupational dose or radiation they receive? There are two methods to measure the levels of radiation and potential exposure to concerned personnel. First, a radiation survey can be performed by a health physicist using ionization chambers to determine radiation levels during exposures at all locations in the office. This type of survey checks the reliability of the x-ray machine and protective barriers. It does not monitor the day-by-day activity of the concerned personnel.

The second method is to have personnel wear pocket dosimeters or film badges. Of the two methods, film badges are less expensive and more widely used. Film badge service is readily available from many radiation survey companies at a nominal monthly cost. The badge (Fig. 2-9) is usually worn for a 3- or 4-week period and contains a film packet, similar to dental film, embossed with the wearer's name and identification number. At the end of the prescribed reporting period, the film packet is returned to the survey company where it is processed; the density on the film is compared with standards and the exposure determined. The report that is returned to the dental office contains not only the exposure for the reporting period but the accumulated quarterly, yearly, and lifetime exposure of the individual. Using the 100 millirem weekly MPD limit, the dental auxiliary's radiation protection can easily be evaluated. The film badge should be worn in the office at all times if it is to be an accurate reading of occupational exposure. If clipped to a pocket it should not be covered with a pen or piece of jewelry that might shield the film. The badge should not be worn outside the office, especially in bright sunlight. The badge should be removed if the person being monitored is to have medical or dental x-rays, because it is intended to measure only occupational exposure.

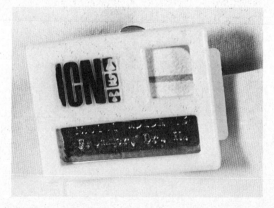

Fig. 2-9. Film badge attached to pocket on operator's uniform. (Courtesy ICN Pharmaceuticals, Inc., Cleveland, Ohio.)

Exposure technique

The dental auxiliary or dentist should never be in the path of the primary beam. Film packets should never be held in the patient's mouth or a drifting tube head held by the person making the exposure. There are no exceptions to this rule. The operator should not make the mistake of saying "I'll just hold the film for the patient this one time." The operator should be a minimum of 6 feet away from the tube head or behind a suitable barrier when the exposure is made. Federal and state regulations require that every x-ray machine be equipped with either a 6-foot retractable exposure cord or a remote switch that will permit such operator positioning. The remote switch is preferable because it prevents lapses in operator technique. Though not as important as distance and shielding, it is important to know where the areas of minimum scatter are. These areas are at right angles to the x-ray beam and toward the back of the patient (Fig. 2-10). The areas of highest scatter are in back of the tube head and behind the patient. Correct positioning of the operator still necessitates the minimum 6-feet distance or adequate barrier protection.

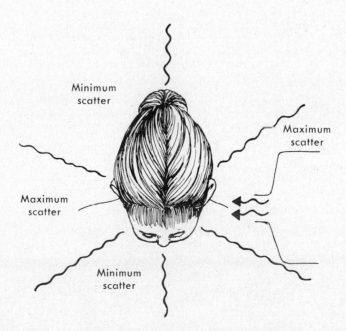

Minimum scatter

Maximum scatter

Maximum scatter

Minimum scatter

Fig. 2-10. Areas of minimum and maximum scatter during dental x-ray exposure.

Shielding

The walls, floor, and ceiling of the x-ray operatory must be of such construction that the surrounding areas will be shielded from both primary and secondary radiation. This does not mean they must be lead-lined. There are many materials used in construction that in the proper thickness will provide protective shielding.

The shielding or barrier requirements are based on such factors as workload, use and occupancy factors, maximum kilovoltage, and distance from the tube head. The formula $W \times U \times T$ is used to calculate the guide number. In this formula W is the work load (in milliampere minutes per week), U is the use factor, and T is the occupancy factor. The guide number is correlated to the proper kVp and distance in reference tables found in Report 35 of the National Committee on Radiation Protection.[15] These tables give the specifications of materials necessary for adequate shielding for the given conditions.

QUALITY ASSURANCE

It is important to establish quality assurance programs in dental offices. The purpose of these programs is to check and monitor x-ray machines, darkroom equipment and procedures, and chairside technique to make sure that ionizing radiation is being used properly and that the maximum diagnostic yield is being achieved for the energy expended. This is an important part of a radiation protection program.

Periodic testing of the performance of the x-ray machine is essential to a program of quality assurance. Some state and local regulatory agencies provide such equipment inspection as part of their registration and licensing program for x-ray machines. The x-ray machines should be checked for timer accuracy, beam quality, collimation, and beam alignment. Quality control in the darkroom involves checks for light leaks, proper safe lighting, strength of processing solutions, condition of film hangers and tanks, accuracy of the thermostat and thermometer, as well as the processing procedure.

Another part of a quality control program is the maintenance of high levels of chairside competence. Using programs of self-evaluation, intraoffice peer review, and continuing education, superior levels of chairside technique can be maintained and retakes kept to a minimum.

STUDY QUESTIONS

1. Explain the difference between the terms exposure and dose.
2. What is the difference between a roentgen, a rad, and a rem?
3. What is a dose response curve? What type is applicable in radiation dosage?
4. What are the major constituents of background radiation?
5. Explain the difference between a localized dose and total body dose.
6. What body cells are most sensitive to ionizing radiation?

7. Approximately what is the facial exposure from a full-mouth x-ray survey? How is it calculated?
8. Explain the "risk vs benefit" concept.
9. What determines selection criteria for dental radiography?
10. Explain what is meant by the maximum permissible dose for dental auxiliaries. What is its present value?
11. What is the present status of administrative radiographs?
12. Where should the dental auxiliary be positioned when taking radiographs?
13. Is it permissible for the dental auxiliary to hold films in handicapped patient's mouth while x-ray exposures are made?
14. What constitutes adequate shielding in the dental office? Are lead walls mandatory?
15. What are the advantages of wearing film badges?

REFERENCES

1. Barnett, M.H.: The biological effects of ionizing radiation, an overview, U.S. Department of Health, Education & Welfare, (F.D.A.) **77**:8004, October 1976.
2. National Academy of Sciences, National Research Council: The biological effects of atomic radiation, Washington, D.C., 1952, The Academy.
3. Richards, A.G.: How hazardous is dental radiography? Oral Surg. **14**:1, January 1961.
4. Greer, D.F.: Determination and analysis of absorbed dose resulting from various intraoral radiographic techniques, Oral Surg. **34**:1, July 1972.
5. Pentel, L.: Current perspectives on radiation, N.Y. J. Dent. **45**:3, March 1975.
6. Budowsky, J., and others: Lack of effect of exposure to radiation during intraoral roentgenographic examination as post examination blood studies, J. Am. Dent. Assoc. **55**:199, August 1957.
7. Nolan, W.E.: Radiation hazards to the patient from oral roentgenography, J. Am. Dent. Assoc. **47**:681, December 1953.
8. White, S.C., and Frey, N.W.: An estimation of somatic hazards to the U.S. population from dental radiography, Oral Surg. **43**:1, January 1977.

9. Performance standards for electronic products: diagnostic x-ray systems and their major components, Fed. Register **37**:16461, 1972.
10. Recommendations in radiographic practices, 1981, Council on Dental Materials, Instruments and Equipment, J. Am. Dent. Assoc. **103**:103, July 1981.
11. Silha, R.A.: The new Kodak Ektaspeed dental x-ray film, Dent. Radiogr. Photogr. **54**(2):32-35, 1981.
12. A summary of recommendations from the Technology Assessment Forum of the National Center for Health Care Technology, J. Am. Dent. Assoc. **103**:423, September 1981.
13. Nowak, A.J., and others: Summary of the Conference on Radiation Exposure in Pediatric Dentistry, J. Am. Dent. Assoc. **103**:426, September 1981.
14. Administratively acquired dental radiographs, U.S. Department of Health and Human Services, September 1981.
15. National Council on Radiation Protection and Measurements: Dental x-ray protection, Report 35, Washington, D.C., 1970, N.C.R.P. Publications.

chapter 3   Intraoral radiographic technique: the paralleling method

THE FULL-MOUTH SURVEY

The full-mouth radiographic survey is one of the cornerstones of a complete oral diagnosis. No dental examination or treatment plan can be considered complete without current or valid radiographs. The full-mouth survey is a difficult procedure to do correctly and requires time and meticulous attention to detail. It bears with it the responsibility of exposing the patient to the least amount of ionizing radiation to obtain the maximum diagnositic yield. Unnecessary radiographs or those of poor quality that have no diagnostic value do not serve the patient's needs and only add to the patient's radiation burden. Whether the radiographs are taken by the dentist or the dental auxiliary is not important, as long as the same standards are maintained.

The full-mouth radiographic survey is usually composed of 14 or more periapical films and, where possible, four bite-wing films. This text will discuss a 15 periapical and four bite-wing film technique, using two films for the maxillary central and lateral incisors. A 14 periapical film series would use one film projection for these four teeth. Some series of more than 15 periapical films include distal maxillary molar projections, anterior bite-wings, and individual radiographs using #1 size film of the six maxillary and four mandibular anterior teeth.

The number of radiographs in a full-mouth survey can be modified to include extra or fewer projections depending on the size of the patient's mouth or tooth position. In all cases, the minimum number of films that satisfy the diagnostic requirements of a full-mouth survey should be used. Film mounts are available in combinations of number and size of film. The radiographic survey should not be determined by the film mount available but by the diagnostic needs of the patient. The recommended film projections (Fig. 3-1) are as follows:

MAXILLARY: Right and left central and lateral incisors
Right and left canines
Right and left premolars
Right and left molars

MANDIBULAR: Central and lateral incisors
Right and left canines
Right and left premolars
Right and left molars

BITE-WING: Right and left premolars
Right and left molars

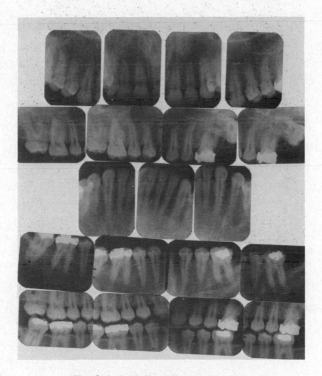

Fig. 3-1. A 19-film full-mouth survey.

A periapical film shows the entire tooth from occlusal edge to apex and 2 to 3 mm of periapical bone. It is this film that is necessary to diagnose normal or pathologic conditions of root, bone, and tooth formation and eruption (Fig. 3-2).

The bite-wing film can be taken only if there are opposing teeth so that the film can be held in position by their occluding surfaces. This film projection shows the upper and lower teeth in occlusion. Only the crown of the teeth are seen. It is used for detecting interproximal decay, periodontal bone loss, recurrent decay under restorations, and the fit of metallic restorations (Fig. 3-3). Bite-wing films can be taken of the anterior teeth but are usually unnecessary.

The full-mouth survey will show all of the teeth in the mandible and maxilla as well as the surrounding bone. Each tooth can be seen at least twice in the survey. That is, the maxillary second premolar can be seen on the premolar periapical film and on the premolar bite-wing film. Some teeth may be seen in three or four views. This gives the diagnostician an opportunity to view the tooth from different radiographic angles and eliminates the possibility of artifact that could be mistaken for caries or other pathologic conditions.

All areas of the jaws are covered in a full-mouth survey. We are not just radiographing the teeth. A clinically edentulous area may have residual root tips, unerupted teeth, or other pathologic conditions in the bone. One should not assume that because there are not teeth present everything is all right. The full complement of periapical films should be taken on all patients.

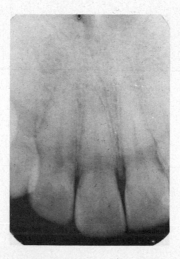

Fig. 3-2. Periapical radiograph of the maxillary central incisor area. Note that the entire tooth and surrounding periapical bone are visualized.

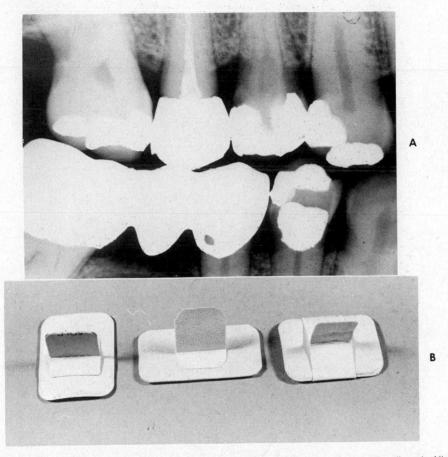

Fig. 3-3. A, Bite-wing radiograph. Note that only the crowns, alveolar ridge, and a small part of the roots of opposing teeth are seen. **B,** Types of bite-wing films: left-vertical, middle-long posterior, and right-standard.

CRITERIA FOR INTRAORAL RADIOGRAPHS

The criteria for judging whether a single radiograph or a full-mouth survey is diagnostically acceptable are:

1. The radiograph should show proper definition and a degree of density and contrast so that all structures can be easily delineated.
2. The structures should not be distorted either by elongation or by foreshortening.
3. The radiograph should show the teeth from the occlusal or incisal edges to 2 to 3 mm beyond their apices.
4. In a full-mouth survey, the entire alveolar processes of the mandible and maxilla must be seen—as far distal as the tuberosity in the maxilla and the beginning of the ascending ramus in the mandible.
5. All interproximal surfaces of the teeth should be seen without overlapping, providing the teeth are not overlapped in the mouth.
6. The x-ray beam should be centered on the film so there are no unexposed parts of the film (''cone cuts,'' or ''collimator cutoff'').
7. The radiograph should not be cracked or bent or have any other artifacts.
8. The radiograph should be processed properly (see Chapter 7).

In a single radiograph, if these criteria have not been met and the radiograph is not diagnostic, then it must be retaken. In a full-mouth survey, it may be possible to see areas and structures that do not appear on the primary film or adjacent films in the series. Although we would like to have a technically perfect full-mouth survey, retakes should not be done unless judged necessary for proper diagnosis.

These criteria should be used to evaluate radiographs taken by dentists and dental auxiliaries as part of a quality assurance program. This can be accomplished by either self-analysis and criticism of one's work or by peer review. In this manner, technical errors will be corrected and high quality diagnostic radiographs produced.

PARALLELING TECHNIQUE

The basic principle of the paralleling technique for intraoral periapical films is that the film packet and the long axis of the tooth being radiographed must be parallel to each other, and the central ray of the x-ray beam must be directed perpendicular to both (see Fig. 1-29). To accomplish this parallelism, the object-film distance must be increased. This distance can be sizable in some areas, such as the maxillary molar projection where the film may have to be held at the midline of the palate to achieve this parallelism.

The increased object-film distance will result in loss of image sharpness and thus is compensated for by using a 16-inch FFD (Fig. 3-4).

Unfortunately, the paralleling technique has too often been called the "long cone technique." This has led to emphasis being placed on the length of the PID rather than on the parallel relationship of the object and the film. Better names for this technique are the "extension paralleling" or "right-angle technique," both of which stress the important components of the technique.

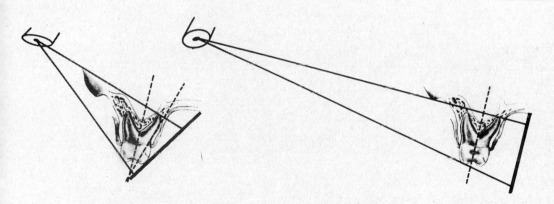

Fig. 3-4. Bisecting, 8-inch focal film distance technique and paralleling 16-inch extended cone technique. Note superimposition of zygomatic arch on apices of maxillary molar in bisecting technique. (Courtesy Rinn Corp., Elgin, Ill.)

Advantages and disadvantages

In discussing the advantages and disadvantages of a technique, one must realize that the advocates of both the bisecting and the paralleling techniques may differ on what they think are the advantages and the disadvantages of each. What one clinician thinks is important may not be as important to another; the final decision on choice of technique in a dental office will probably be determined by the personal preference of the practitioner. This text takes the position that the paralleling technique is the method of choice.

Advantages of the paralleling technique compared to the bisecting technique. The major advantage of the paralleling technique is that when performed correctly, the image formed on the film will have both linear and dimensional accuracy and the diagnosis made from the radiograph will be more valid. The key terms are dimensional accuracy and dimensional distortion.

The bisecting technique will represent the teeth correct linearly but will have dimensional distortion. The bisecting technique projects the images of the teeth and surrounding structures on the film in a true linear relationship without elongation or foreshortening. A tooth 22 mm in length, when radiographed with the bisecting technique, will be seen on the radiograph as 22 mm long. The teeth and bone, however, are three

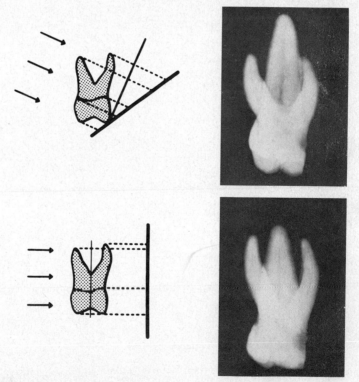

Fig. 3-5. Radiographs of maxillary molar taken with bisecting technique *(top)* and the paralleling technique *(bottom)*. (Courtesy Rinn Corp., Elgin, Ill.)

dimensional objects, and although their overall length may be recorded accurately, the relationship of one part of the tooth to another will be dimensionally distorted (Fig. 3-5). Those parts of the tooth that lie farthest from the film, for example, the buccal plate of bone and buccal roots, will be foreshortened although their lingual linear counterparts will not. The classic clinical example of this is comparing the length of the buccal roots to palatal roots in maxillary first molars. Those clinicians who have used the bisecting technique for many years may really come to believe that the buccal roots are much shorter than they really are because of dimensional distortions. One may argue that this may not be clinically important, except in an initial endodontic measurement, but when this distortion is applied to periodontal evaluation of alveolar bone levels, the clinical importance becomes apparent (Fig. 3-6). In the bisecting technique the image of the buccal bone level is figuratively added to the palatal bone height to give a distorted image.

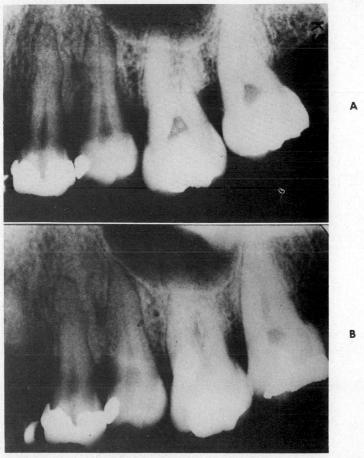

A

B

Fig. 3-6. Radiographs of the same area taken with the paralleling technique, **A,** and the bisecting technique, **B.** Note the difference in alveolar bone height.

A diagnosis could then be made of adequate bone for restorations, splinting, etc. on distorted radiographic images.

With the paralleling technique it is possible to diagnose and evaluate caries and alveolar bone height accurately on all radiographs and not rely on the bite-wing projections, like the users of the bisecting technique do. It is interesting to note that bite-wing projections in both techniques are paralleling films.

In the bisecting technique the radiopaque image of the zygomatic arch is often superimposed upon the apices of the maxillary molars, making diagnosis very difficult if not impossible. This superimposition is understandable because the point of entry of the central ray for molar projections is along the zygomatic arch.

In the paralleling technique there is no superimposition, since the central ray, which is perpendicular to the long axis of the molars, enters below the level of the zygomatic arch (see Fig. 3-4).

The paralleling technique is easier to standardize than the bisecting technique and serial comparison radiographs of the same area have greater validity. This is especially important in evaluating alveolar bone levels of periodontal patients in recall examinations.

If the film-holding device used has a localizing ring, the patient does not have to be positioned so that the occlusal plane of the jaw being radiographed is parallel to the floor. This is especially helpful in contour chairs or where patients are treated in the supine position.

Disadvantages. One of the objections most often raised in regard to the paralleling technique is the difficulty in placing and the degree of discomfort caused by the devices used to hold the film parallel to the long axis of the tooth. In patients with small mouths, children, and patients with low palatal vaults this may present some problems, but the more adept one becomes with the technique the less these problems are a factor.

It is said that paralleling is more difficult to learn and takes clinically longer to do. Experience with novice auxiliary students has proved this to be incorrect. At the least, the time element is the same and learning the paralleling technique is as easy or easier than learning the bisecting technique.

Objections have been raised to the "long bulky" 16 inch extension cylinder that is used in the paralleling technique. It is claimed that it is difficult to work with in small operatories. The difference is 8 inches and this objection has no validity in the newer x-ray machines with the extended FFD within the tube head (see Fig. 1-11).

Another supposed disadvantage of the paralleling technique is that with the 16-inch FFD longer exposure times are necessary and there may be greater chance of patient movement. With the use of faster film this is no longer true. We are comparing exposure times of $\frac{1}{5}$ vs $\frac{4}{5}$ second (inverse square law) and the difference in the possible patient movement within these time frames is not significant. Previously, with the use of slower film the possibility of patient movement with a 4-second exposure, compared to a 1-second exposure, was greater and the objection was valid.

EXPOSURE ROUTINE

Regardless of which technique is used, there are certain basic rules that must be followed regarding personal cleanliness, preparation of the patient, and radiation hygiene. A routine should be developed so that mistakes that necessitate retaking of films can be avoided. Retaking a radiograph because of an error on the part of an operator adds unnecessarily to the patient's radiation burden.

The patient should be seated comfortably in the chair, with his back well supported and his head positioned so that the jaw can be radiographed correctly. Except when localizing rings are used, the occlusal plane of the jaw being radiographed should be parallel to the floor when it is in the open position.

The patient should remove any nonfixed prosthetic appliances from his mouth, as well as eyeglasses from his face. Failure to do this is a common error. Glass and any metallic frame are radiopaque and may be superimposed on the film in the maxillary canine and premolar areas.

The patient should be draped with a lead apron. This is done routinely on all patients, for a single film as well as the full-mouth series. The x-ray machine should then be turned on and the desired kilovoltage and milliamperage selected.

At this point, the operator's hands should be washed. An intraoral procedure is about to be performed, and clean hands are necessary.

Most dental offices will have a semiautomatic lead film dispenser in each operatory. This enables the operator to withdraw one film at a time. The exposed films are placed in a lead receptacle. If there is no lead dispenser, the desired number of films, as well as additional supplies such as bite-wing tabs and bite blocks, should be brought near the operatory at this time.

If there are no lead film dispenser and exposed-film receptacle, both the exposed and unexposed films must be kept out of the room where the x-ray machine is being used. Many diagnostic dental films are fogged and thus made unacceptable because they are left on the bracket table in the dental operatory when other films are being exposed. Again, poor technique on the part of the operator leads to film retakes and unnecessary exposure for the patient.

One of the more important general principles of intraoral radiography is to have the positioned film in the patient's mouth for as little time as possible. This will decrease the likelihood of gagging and patient movement. The desired exposure time on the machine should always be set before placing the film in the patient's mouth. Many seconds can be wasted in consulting exposure charts and setting the timing dial while the film is in the patient's mouth.

While making the exposure from the required 6-foot distance the patient should be watched. In this way, if the patient moves, the error will be detected and a retake film can be done immediately. A properly designed office will permit this observation.

After the exposure has been made, the film is removed from the patient's mouth, dried of saliva, and placed in the exposed-film receptacle.

75

In taking a full-mouth series of radiographs some definite order should be followed. Skipping from area to area without a set pattern will always result in an omitted film. This textbook recommends starting with the maxillary central incisor film. This film is probably the easiest to position and easiest for the patient to tolerate. One should never start with the maxillary molar film because this is the projection most likely to excite the gag reflex; once the reflex is excited, the patient may gag on films that could normally be tolerated. After starting with the maxillary central incisor, the maxillary canine, premolar, and molar are radiographed in that order. The opposite side of the maxilla is then radiographed. It is poor technique to radiograph left canine, right canine, left premolar, and so forth. This necessitates moving the tube head constantly from one side of the patient to the other and usually results in an omitted film.

The bite-wing films are taken after maxillary periapicals since the same head position and occlusal plane orientation are used. The mandibular periapical films are then taken in the same order that the maxillary films were taken.

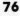

METHOD

In the paralleling technique the film packet may be held in its proper position by a variety of devices all serving one purpose: to keep the long axis of the film parallel to the long axis of the tooth. Some of the devices, such as cotton rolls, hemostats, bite blocks, XCP, and Precision holders are pictured in Fig. 3-7. Localizing rings, which align the cone with the film in both the horizontal and the vertical planes, are shown attached to the XCP and Precision devices. The localizing rings are a great aid in some of the contour dental chairs in which it may be difficult to position the patient so that the occlusal plane is parallel to the floor. As long as the open-ended PID can be brought into flat contact with the localizing ring, strict adherence to occlusal plane orientation is not necessary.

There are factors that must be considered in any periapical projection: exposure time, chair position, film position and placement, point of entry of the beam, vertical angulation, and horizontal angulation.

Exposure time. Exposure time is determined by the area being radiographed, the film speed, kVp, milliamperage, and FFD. Exposure charts are readily available, and most x-ray film packages contain them. It is customary to post such a chart near the machine so the exposure times need not be committed to memory. Exposure times should be set before placing the film in the patient's mouth.

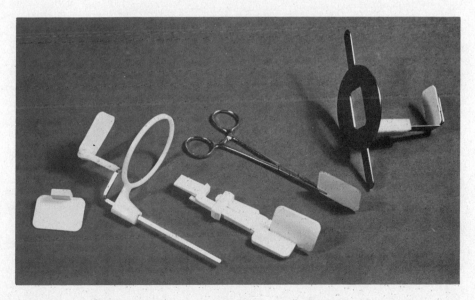

Fig. 3-7. Film-holding devices for use in paralleling technique. Left to right: bite block, XCP and localizing ring, Snap-a-Ray, hemostat, Precision paralleling device.

Chair position — occlusal and sagittal plane orientations. The patient is positioned so that when the mouth is open and the film packet is in position, the occusal plane of the jaw being radiographed is parallel to the floor. In the maxilla this plane corresponds to the ala-tragus line on the face. When the maxilla is radiographed, the headrest is positioned high on the back of the patient's head, forcing the chin down (Fig. 3-8). When the mandible is filmed, the headrest is placed below the occipital eminence, in what would be the normal dental chair position (Fig. 3-9). For both upper and lower jaws the patient's head is positioned so that the sagittal plane is perpendicular to the floor (Fig. 3-10).

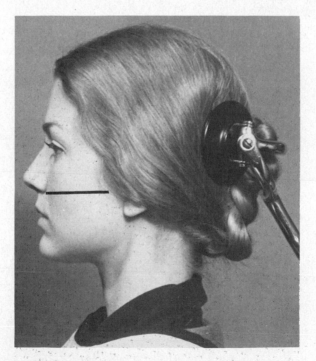

Fig. 3-8. Proper patient position for maxillary periapical radiographs and bite-wing films. Note that occlusal plane of maxillary teeth, or ala-tragus line, is parallel to the floor.

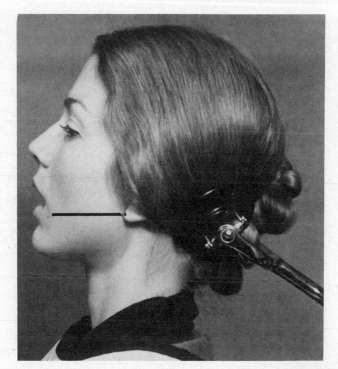

Fig. 3-9. Proper patient position for mandibular periapical radiographs. Note that when mouth is open occlusal plane of lower teeth is parallel to the floor.

Fig. 3-10. Proper patient position for orientation of sagittal plane of head perpendicular to the floor.

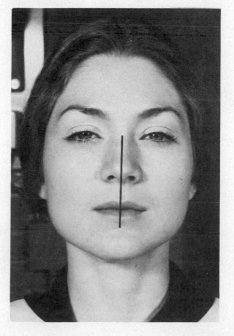

Film position. The film packet is held with its long dimension vertical for anterior projections and horizontal for posterior periapical and bite-wing projections. The edge of the film should always extend evenly either ⅛ inch below (maxillary) or above (mandibular) the occlusal plane. This ensures adequate film at the apical area to record the image. The film should be placed in the patient's mouth with the operator's thumb and forefinger so that the mounting orientation button is toward the occlusal surface (Fig. 3-11). This helps in mounting and precludes the possibility of the dot being superimposed over the apex of a tooth. The film is held in position by the patient with either a finger, bite block, or other positioning device.

Point of entry. Point of entry is the anatomic position on the patient's face at which the central ray of the x-ray beam is aimed. It corresponds to the middle of the film packet in the patient's mouth. The operator should know these anatomic points but should also align the beam with the film as viewed in the patient's mouth.

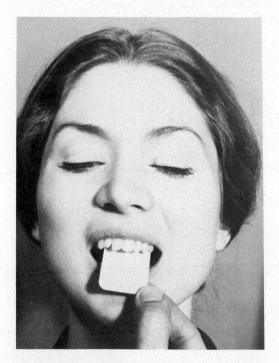

Fig. 3-11. Placement of film packet in patient's mouth by operator's thumb and forefinger. Note that correct side of film packet faces tube head and mounting dot is toward incisal edge.

80

Vertical angulation. In the paralleling technique the vertical angulation is set to make the central ray perpendicular to the film. In the bisecting technique the vertical angulation is determined by the bisection of the angle. The vertical angulation given in this text and elsewhere should be used only as guide angles. With ideal film positioning these angles can be strictly adhered to. Not all mouths will allow this type of film positioning. Some mouths have crowded arches, misplaced teeth, and tight muscle attachments. In these cases, the bisection of the film-tooth angle will result in different vertical angulations than the ones listed. Vertical angulation of the x-ray beam is set according to the dial on the side of the tube head (Fig. 3-12).

Horizontal angulation. The central ray is directed so that it is perpendicular to the film in the horizontal plane. It can also be said that the central ray is directed through the interproximal spaces to avoid overlapping of structures. It may be easier for the operator to sight on the horizontal axis of the tube head and make this parallel to the film in the horizontal plane.

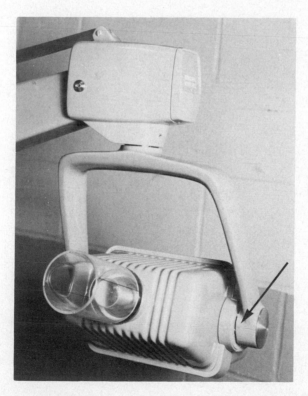

Fig. 3-12. Photograph of tube head of x-ray machine, with arrow pointing to setting for vertical angulation.

THE FULL-MOUTH SERIES

Maxillary central and lateral incisors (Fig. 3-13)

Chair position. The maxillary occlusal plane is positioned parallel to the floor, and the sagittal plane of the patient's face is perpendicular to the floor.

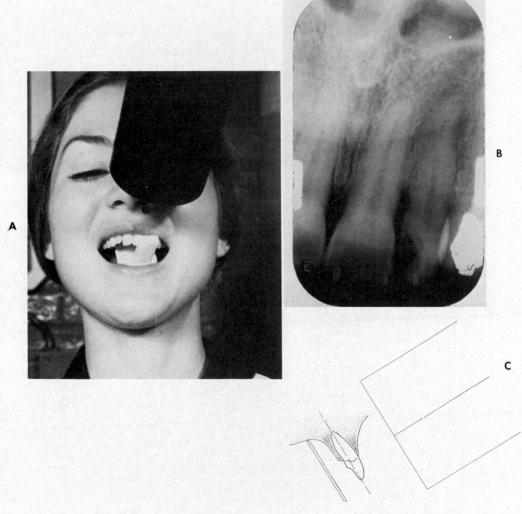

Fig. 3-13. Maxillary central and lateral incisors. **A,** Film packet and position-indicating device (PID). Dot represents point of entry of central ray. **B,** Radiograph. **C,** Diagram.

Film position. The film is held vertically and positioned in the palate away from the lingual surfaces of the teeth so that the long axis of the film packet will be parallel to the long axis of the teeth. The center of the film packet is between the central and lateral incisors. The film is positioned in the palate so that the entire length of the teeth will be shown. This parallel placement of the film is held in position by one of the devices previously mentioned.

Point of entry. The central ray is directed at the center of the film. If a localizing ring is used, the open face of the PID contacts the ring; this will then determine the point of entry and vertical and horizontal angulation of the x-ray beam.

Vertical angulation. The central ray is perpendicular to the film packet.

Horizontal angulation. The central ray is perpendicular to the film in the horizontal plane.

If one film is to be used for the maxillary right and left central and lateral incisors, the center of the film is placed between the central incisors and the central ray is directed perpendicular to the center of the film packet (Fig. 3-14).

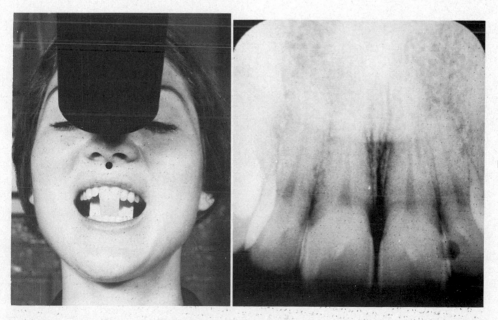

Fig. 3-14. Right and left maxillary central and lateral incisors. **A,** Film packet and PID. Dot represents point of entry. **B,** Radiograph.

Maxillary canines (Fig. 3-15)

Chair position. The maxillary occlusal plane is parallel to the floor, and the sagittal plane of the patient's face is perpendicular to the floor.

Film position. The film is held vertically, away from the lingual surface of the canine, and parallel to its long axis. The center of the film packet is behind the canine and is positioned in the palate so that the entire length of the canine will be shown. The film packet is held in position by some previously mentioned device.

Point of entry. The central ray is directed at the center of the film packet, or if localizing ring is used, it is brought into flat contact with the open-ended PID.

Vertical angulation. The central ray is perpendicular to the film packet.

Horizontal angulation. The central ray is perpendicular to the film in the horizontal plane.

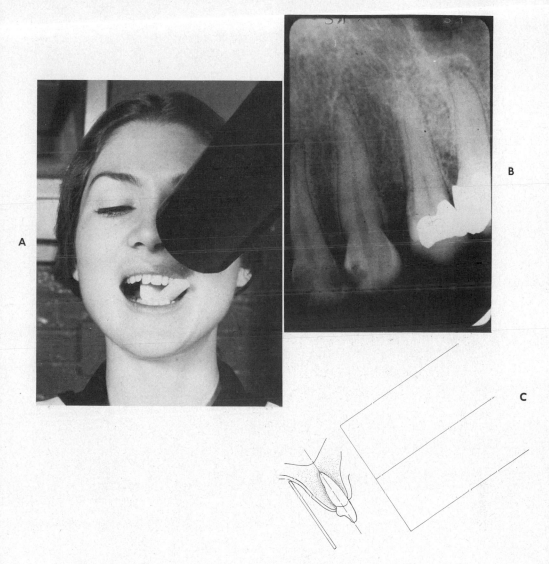

Fig. 3-15. Maxillary canine. **A,** Film packet and PID. **B,** Radiograph. **C,** Diagram.

Maxillary premolars (Fig. 3-16)

Chair position. The maxillary occlusal plane is parallel to the floor, and the sagittal plane of the patient's face is perpendicular to the floor.

Film position. The film is held horizontally and positioned away from the lingual surfaces of the premolar so that its long axis is parallel to the long axis of the premolar. In the maxillary premolar and molar region this may position the film in the middle of the palate. The center of the film aligns with the second premolar. The packet is positioned in the palate so that the entire length of the teeth will be shown on the film. The packet is held in position by some previously mentioned device.

Point of entry. The central ray is directed at the center of the film, or if a localizing ring is used it is brought into flat contact with the open-ended PID.

Vertical angulation. The central ray is perpendicular to the film.

Horizontal angulation. The central ray is perpendicular to the film in the horizontal plane.

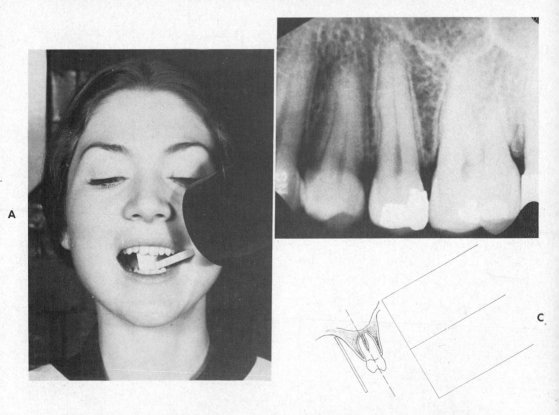

Fig. 3-16. Maxillary premolars. **A,** Film packet and PID. **B,** Radiograph. **C,** Diagram.

Maxillary molars (Fig. 3-17)

Chair position. The maxillary occlusal plane is positioned parallel to the floor, and the sagittal plane of the patient's face is perpendicular to the floor.

Film position. The film is held horizontally and positioned away from the lingual surfaces of the molars so that the long axis of the film will be parallel to the long axes of the molars. The center of the film packet aligns to the middle of the second molar, and the packet is positioned in the palate so the entire length of the teeth will be shown. The film packet is held in position by some previously mentioned device.

Point of entry. The central ray is directed at the center of the film, or the localizing ring is brought into flat contact with the open-ended PID.

Vertical angulation. The central ray is perpendicular to the film.

Horizontal angulation. The central ray is perpendicular to the film in the horizontal plane.

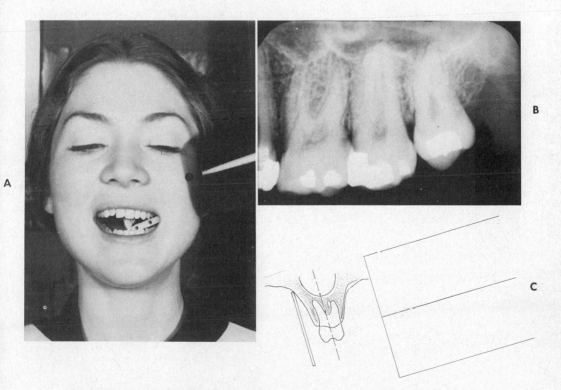

Fig. 3-17. Maxillary molars. **A,** Film packet and PID. **B,** Radiograph. **C,** Diagram.

BITE-WING FILMS

The technique for bite-wing films is the same in the paralleling and bisecting-angle technique except for the use of the 16-inch FFD and thus increased exposure time. Bite-wing films are always parallel films no matter what technique is used for the periapical films. The film is positioned by the bite tab parallel to the crowns of both upper and lower teeth, and the central ray is directed perpendicular to the film.

Premolar and molar bite-wing projections (Fig. 3-18)

Chair position. The maxillary occlusal plane is positioned parallel to the floor, and the sagittal plane of the patient's face is perpendicular to the floor.

Film position. When the premolars are radiographed, the bite tab is placed on the occlusal surfaces of the first and second mandibular premolars. This will depress the film packet into the floor of the mouth. While the operator holds the tab down with thumb and forefinger, the patient is instructed to bite on the tab. The operator should be sure that the patient is biting on the back teeth and not just bringing the incisors together. If the back teeth are not moved to centric occlusion, the film packet will not be oriented correctly. The procedure for radiographing the molars is the same as that previously mentioned except that the bite tab is centered over the occlusal surface of the second molar.

Point of entry. The central ray is directed at the bite-wing tab, which is held in position by the patient's teeth.

Vertical angulation. $+10°$.

Horizontal angulation. Horizontal angulation is a critical factor in the bite-wing film, and utmost attention should be paid to horizontal position. An overlapping image on the bite-wing film is useless. The central ray should be perpendicular to the film packet in the horizontal plane and should go through the contact points of the premolars or molars.

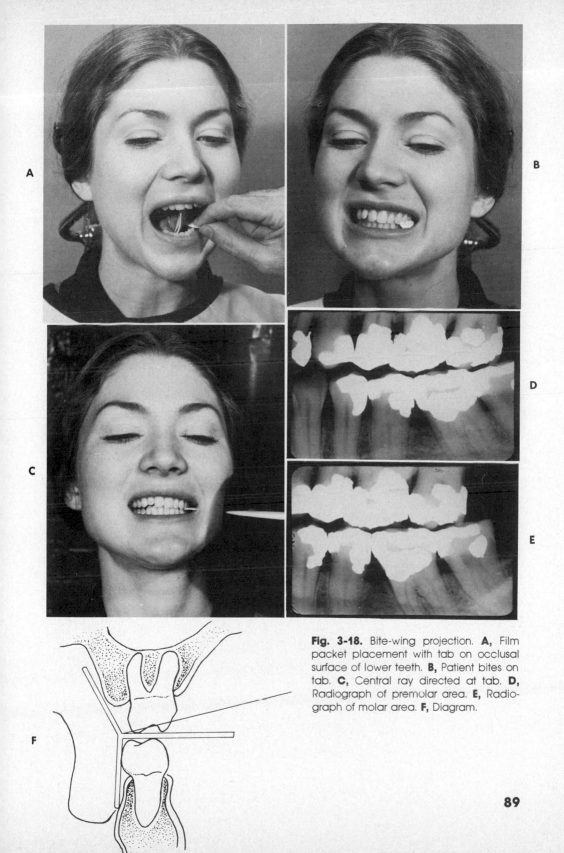

Fig. 3-18. Bite-wing projection. **A,** Film packet placement with tab on occlusal surface of lower teeth. **B,** Patient bites on tab. **C,** Central ray directed at tab. **D,** Radiograph of premolar area. **E,** Radiograph of molar area. **F,** Diagram.

89

VERTICAL BITE-WINGS (Fig. 3-19)

Vertical bite-wings are used when the desired area would not be seen on the film with normal bite-wing placement; this could be the case in advanced bone loss or root caries. The film is placed in the patient's mouth with the longer side vertically positioned. All other exposure factors remain the same. It is necessary to use the paste-on tabs and not the loops or the preformed bite-wing packets in this technique.

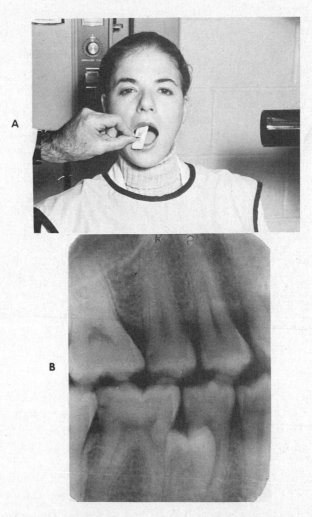

Fig. 3-19. Vertical bite-wing. **A,** Film position. **B,** Radiograph.

Mandibular incisors (Fig. 3-20)

Chair position. The patient is positioned so that when the mouth is open the mandibular occlusal plane is parallel to the floor, and the sagittal plane of the patient's face is perpendicular to the floor.

Film position. The film is held vertically and positioned away from the lingual surfaces of the incisors so that the long axis of the film will be parallel to the long axes of the incisors. The center of the packet is positioned at the midline so that all four incisors will appear on the film. The film is depressed into the floor of the mouth so that the entire length of the teeth will be shown. It may be necessary to displace the tongue distally as well as to depress the floor of the mouth to achieve this. The film packet is held in position by some previously mentioned device.

Point of entry. The central ray is directed at the center of the film, or the localizing ring is brought into flat contact with the open-ended PID.

Vertical angulation. The central ray is perpendicular to the film.

Horizontal angulation. The central ray is perpendicular to the film in the horizontal plane.

Fig. 3-20. Mandibular incisors. **A,** Film packet and PID. **B,** Radiograph. **C,** Diagram.

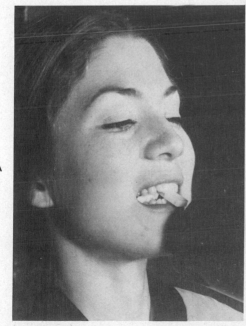

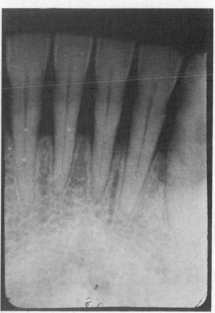

B

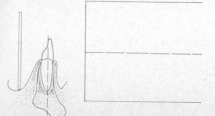

C

Mandibular canines (Fig. 3-21)

Chair position. The patient is positioned so that when the mouth is open the mandibular occlusal plane is parallel to the floor, and the sagittal plane of the patient's face is perpendicular to the floor.

Film position. The film is held vertically and positioned away from the lingual surface of the canine so that its long axis will be parallel to that of the canine. The packet is positioned so that the canine will be in the center of the film. The packet is depressed into the floor of the mouth so that the entire length of the teeth will be shown on the film. The packet is held in position by some previously mentioned device.

Point of entry. The central ray is directed at the center of the film, or the localizing ring is brought into flat contact with the open-ended PID.

Vertical angulation. The central ray is perpendicular to the film.

Horizontal angulation. The central ray is perpendicular to the film in the horizontal plane.

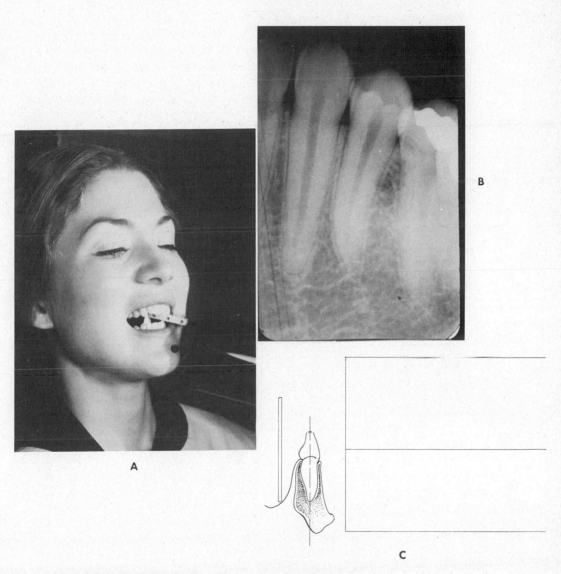

Fig. 3-21. Mandibular canine. **A,** Film packet and PID. **B,** Radiograph. **C,** Diagram.

Mandibular premolars (Fig. 3-22)

Chair position. The patient is positioned so that when the mouth is open the mandibular occlusal plane is parallel to the floor, and the sagittal plane of the patient's face is perpendicular to the floor.

Film position. The film is held horizontally and positioned so that it is parallel to the long axes of the premolar. The object-film distance in both the mandibular premolar and molar regions is almost minimum since the anatomy allows the film to be positioned very close to the tooth and still be parallel. The second premolar is centered behind the center of the film packet. The packet is depressed into the floor of the mouth so that the entire length of the teeth will show on the film. The film is held in position by some previously mentioned device.

Point of entry. The central ray is directed at the center of the film, or if a localizing ring is used, it is brought into flat contact with the open-ended PID.

Vertical angulation. The central ray is directed perpendicular to the film.

Horizontal angulation. The central ray is perpendicular to the film in the horizontal plane.

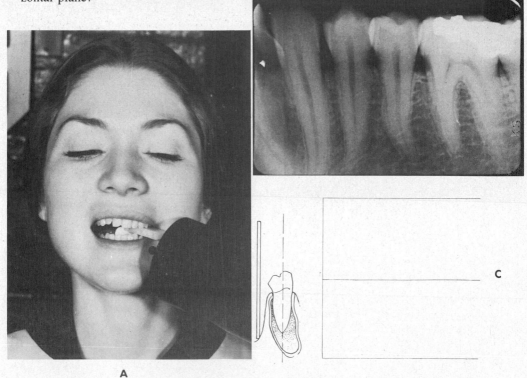

A

B

C

Fig. 3-22. Mandibular premolar. **A,** Film packet and PID. **B,** Radiograph. **C,** Diagram.

Mandibular molars (Fig. 3-23)

Chair position. The patient is positioned so that when the mouth is open the mandibular occlusal plane is parallel to the floor, and the sagittal plane of the patient's face is perpendicular to the floor.

Film position. The film is held horizontally and positioned lingually to the molar so that the long axis of the film is parallel to the long axes of the molars. The film is centered behind the second molar and depressed into the floor of the mouth so that the entire length of the teeth will appear on the film. The packet is held in position by some previously mentioned device.

Point of entry. The central ray is directed at the center of the film, or if a localizing ring is used, it is brought into flat contact with the open-ended PID.

Vertical angulation. The central ray is directed perpendicular to the film.

Horizontal angulation. The central ray is perpendicular to the film in the horizontal plane.

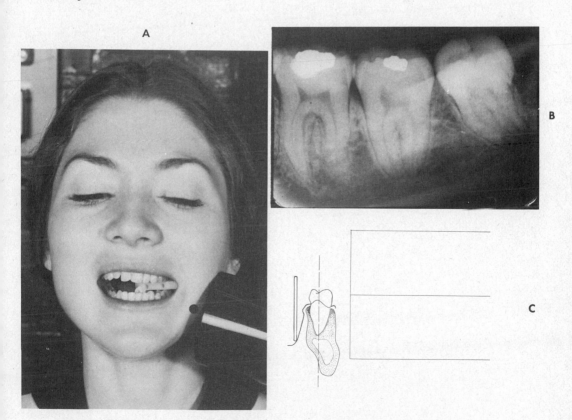

Fig. 3-23. Mandibular molars. **A,** Film packet and PID. **B,** Radiograph. **C,** Diagram.

95

COMMON ERRORS

All the errors mentioned and illustrated in this chapter are also possible in the bisecting technique, but the incidence differs. Whereas elongation and foreshortening are the most common bisecting errors, they are not that common in the paralleling technique. The most common error in the paralleling technique, even with the use of positioning devices, is film placement. If the film packet and positioning device are not placed correctly in the patient's mouth, the paralleling technique will not work. The most common error is to not place the film packet deep enough in the floor of the mouth or high enough in the palate, thus cutting off the apices of the teeth.

With the use of the localizing ring, which is aligned with the center of the film packet, "cone cutting" can be practically eliminated.

Occlusal plane and sagittal plane orientation of the patient's head is not important if the localizing ring on the film-holding device is used, as long as the open end of the cylinder is brought into flat contact with the localizing ring.

Horizontal overlapping of the images is also eliminated with the proper use of the positioning device and localizing ring.

The rest of the errors mentioned in this chapter (that is, film reversal, overbending, crescent marks, overexposing and underexposing, double exposure, and failure to remove dental appliances) are all possible with the bisecting technique, and their remedies are the same.

Cone cutting (collimator cutoff) (Fig. 3-24)

An unexposed area on the radiograph occurs when the x-ray beam is not centered on the film packet. This is called "cone cutting" and is caused by improper x-ray beam film alignment.

Remedy. Carefully align the central ray of the x-ray beam with the center of the film packet. With circular collimation the aperture of the diaphragm allows for a beam diameter, measured at the face, of 2¾ inches. Size #2 adult film is 1¼ × 1⅝ inches, which leaves almost ½ inch leeway for error in all directions. It is not sufficient to identify collimator cutoff; it should be analyzed to pinpoint the error. If it is always the distal part of a radiograph in a projection that is cut off, then the point of entry must be moved mesially. A localizing ring, with a film-holding device, will align the beam and the film and eliminate collimator cutoff.

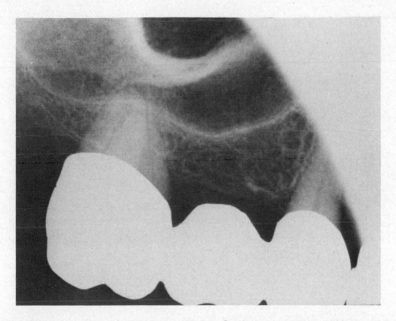

Fig. 3-24. Collimator cutoff ("cone cutting"). Central ray positioned too far distal.

Film reversal (Fig. 3-25)

Film reversal is sometimes referred to as the "herringbone effect" because the herringbone pattern embossed on the lead foil backing is transferred to the processed, reversed radiograph. The "herringbone" light film results from placing the film packet backward in the patient's mouth. The x-rays are attenuated by the lead foil before striking the film. The pattern embossed in the lead that appears on the film distinguishes this light film from other underexposure errors.

Remedy. Always note the front and back of the film packet. Some manufacturers color code or change the texture of the back of the packet. Develop the habit of looking for these aids.

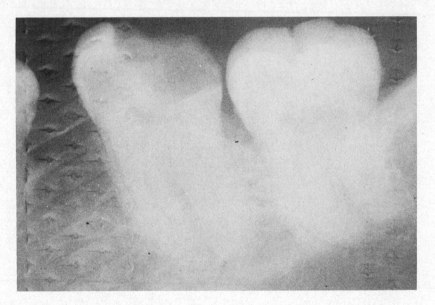

Fig. 3-25. Film reversal. Film packet placed in mouth with the wrong side toward the tube.

Film placement (Fig. 3-26)

The film has been poorly positioned if the whole tooth does not show on the film and the image is not elongated; there is no film behind the apex of the tooth to record the image.

Remedy. Make sure there is only ⅛ inch of film projecting above or below the occlusal or incisal edges of the teeth. If a bite block is used, the teeth being radiographed must be biting firmly on the block.

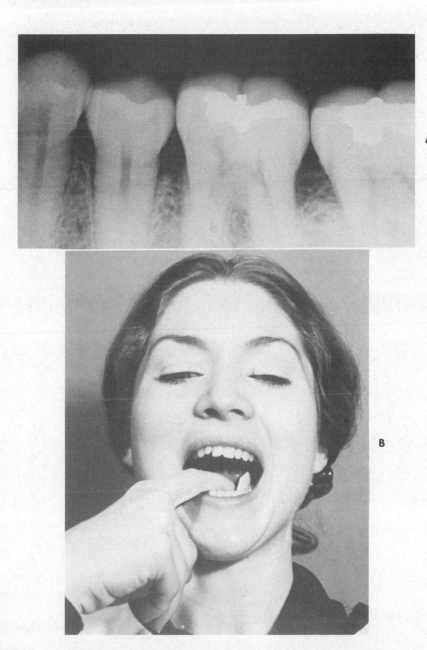

A

B

Fig. 3-26. A, Nondiagnostic radiograph due to poor film-packet placement. Note that apices of teeth are not seen. **B,** Poor film placement. Note how much film is visible above occlusal plane of tooth.

Overlapping (Figs. 3-27 and 3-28)

Overlapping of the images of the teeth will result if the central ray is not perpendicular to the film and teeth in the horizontal plane.

Remedy. Align the film with some part of the tube head that is perpendicular to the central ray. There is usually a horizontal bar with the manufacturer's name on it. Stand in front of the patient, retract the patient's cheek, and check the horizontal alignment. As in film reversal, a positioning device with a localizing ring can be used to prevent overlapping. If the film is placed parallel to the teeth, the localizing ring will align the beam perpendicular to the film.

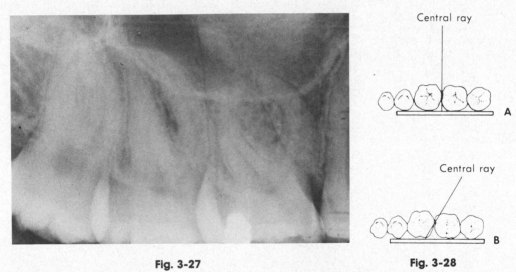

Fig. 3-27   **Fig. 3-28**

Fig. 3-27. Overlapped images.
Fig. 3-28. A, Proper and **B,** improper horizontal angulation of x-ray beam.

Crescent marks and bent films (Figs. 3-29 and 3-30)

Black crescent-shaped marks can be caused by excessive bending of the film packet, which cracks the emulsion. The crescent marks show when the film is developed. A film may be overbent to such a degree that the x-rays will not strike it at all.

Remedy. Films can be made more pliable by rolling them slightly against one's index finger, which also may allow them to fit better in the patient's mouth. Films should not be bent to adapt to anatomic surfaces. X-rays travel in straight lines; they do not turn corners to expose bent films.

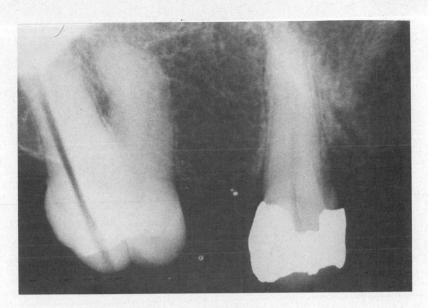

Fig. 3-29. Black line due to cracking of film emulsion.

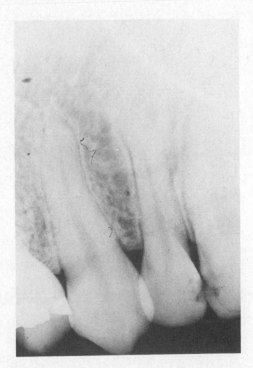

Fig. 3-30. Result of over bending film packet. Note upper right corner.

Light films (Fig. 3-31)

Light films or films that do not have enough density can result from underexposure or underdevelopment, assuming that the proper kVp has been used. If enough kVp has not been used, the dental structures will be underpenetrated and the film, although light, will not differentiate structures of different density.

Remedy. Underexposure—check all settings on the machine before making an exposure (mA, time, kVp).

A very common error that leads to underexposure is unwittingly increasing the FFD. This is done by failing to bring the open end of the cylinder close to the patient's face. The exposure times are calculated for an FFD that assumes a cylinder placement close to the face. If the cylinder is carelessly positioned away from the face, the inverse square law will intensify the error, not just by the increased distance but the square of that distance (Fig. 3-32). Underdevelopment—see Chapter 7.

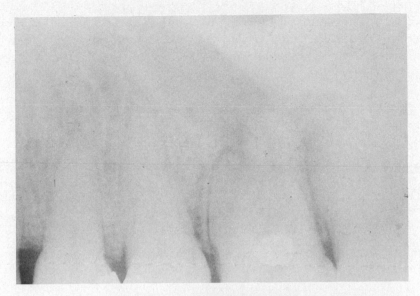

Fig. 3-31. Underexposed radiograph.

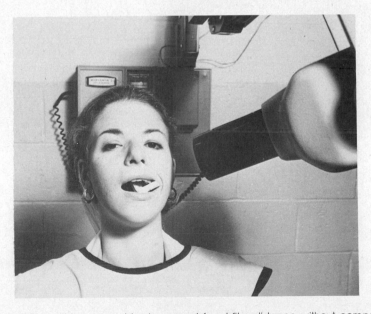

Fig. 3-32. Light film will be caused by increased focal-film distance without compensatory increase in exposure time. Note distance between patient's face and PID.

Dark film (Fig. 3-33)

Dark film is caused by overexposure or overdevelopment, the reverse causes of light films. The length of the PID prevents the possibility of decreased FFD. If a film is overpenetrated, it will be black and none of the dental structures will show or they will be difficult to differentiate.

Remedy. Overexposure—check all settings on the control panel before making an exposure. Overdevelopment—see Chapter 6.

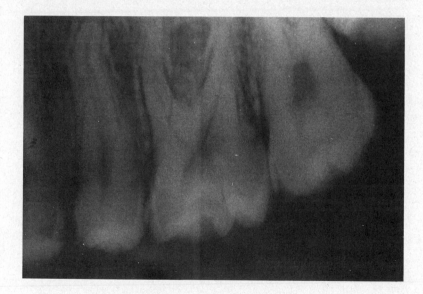

Fig. 3-33. Overexposed radiograph.

Double exposure (Fig. 3-34)

A double exposure results from using the same film packet twice. This is an unforgivable error and indicates lack of attention to detail.

Remedy. After the film packet has been exposed, place it in a lead receptacle. Never keep the exposed and unexposed films on the same shelf.

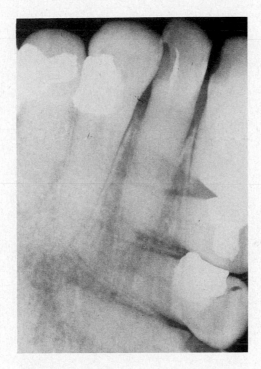

Fig. 3-34. Double exposure on radiograph.

Blurred images (Fig. 3-35)

Blurred images are the result of either patient, film, or tube head movement during the exposure.

Remedy. Adjust tube heads and arms to prevent vibration and drifting. Good chairside technique will prevent film and patient movement.

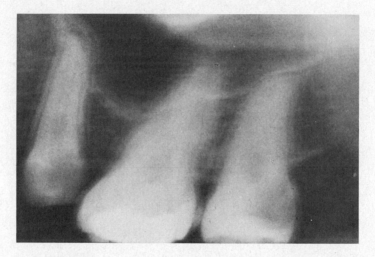

Fig. 3-35. Blurred image caused by patient movement.

Failure to remove dental appliances (Fig. 3-36)

If dental appliances are not removed the metallic portions will be superimposed on the tooth structure.

Remedy. Make it part of the work routine to have patients remove all dentures and eyeglasses. For panoramic and extraoral projections patients must also remove earrings, hearing aids, and hair clips.

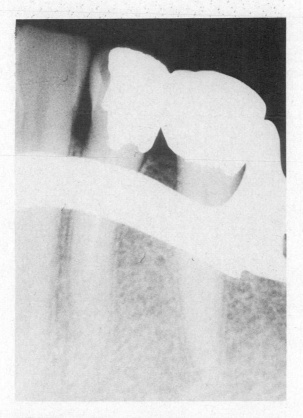

Fig. 3-36. Patient's partial denture was not removed.

Poor bite-wings (Fig. 3-37)

The three most common errors seen on bite-wing radiographs are overlapping, collimator cutoff, and film placement.

Overlapping (Fig. 3-37, *A*). Overlapping is a result of improper horizontal beam alignment.

Remedy. Align the beam in the horizontal plane so that it is at right angles to the film packet.

Collimator cutoff – "cone cutting" (Fig. 3-37, *B*). Collimator cutoff is failure to align the central ray with the center of the film packet. It occurs most often because the operator loses sight of the bite tab when the patient closes the mouth.

Remedy. Keep the bite tab visible by asking the patient to smile while biting. If this is not possible, touch the tab with one hand while aligning the beam with the other. The central ray is directed at the tab (Fig. 3-38).

Poor film placement (see Fig. 3-37, *C*). Poor film placement occurs in bite-wing films when either the patient is allowed to bite the film into position after the operator has let go of the tab or the patient bites in protrusive instead of centric relation, allowing the film to float free and be repositioned by the tongue.

Remedy. Do not let go of the film tab until the patient is biting on it in centric occlusion.

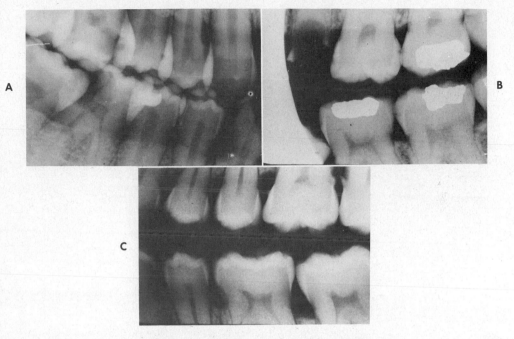

Fig. 3-37. A, Overlapped bite-wing. **B,** Collimator cutoff on bite-wing. **C,** Improper film placement.

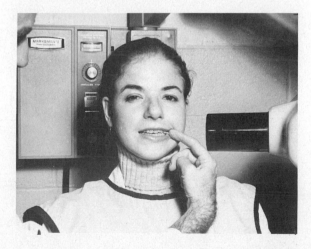

Fig. 3-38. Aligning the x-ray beam with the bite-wing tab by seeing the tab and/or touching it.

109

STUDY QUESTIONS

1. Explain dimensional distortion and how it applies to the paralleling technique.
2. What is the advantage of an increased FFD (8 to 16 inches)?
3. What is parallel in the paralleling technique?
4. What is a localizing ring and what is its function?
5. Name some devices that can be used to hold film in the paralleling technique.
6. What is the size of the x-ray beam as it reaches the face in the paralleling technique?
7. Why is the paralleling technique superior to the bisecting technique in interpreting periodontal bone height?
8. Why is there no superimposition of the zygomatic arch on the apices of maxillary molars in the paralleling technique?
9. Can the paralleling technique be used with an 8-inch FFD?
10. What technique is always used in the bite-wing projection?

chapter 4 Bisecting technique, edentulous and pedodontic surveys

In the bisecting technique, the film packet is placed as close to the tooth as possible without bending the film. Because of the anatomy of the mouth, the long axis of the tooth will not be parallel to the plane of the film with this placement. The vertical angulation of the tube head is directed so that the central ray will be perpendicular to a line that bisects the angle formed by the long axis of the tooth and the plane of the dental film (see Fig. 1-30). With this film placement, the object-film distance is at a minmum. No compensation for image enlargement is necessary and the technique usually calls for an 8-inch FFD. Although a "short cone" is used, this is not the determining factor in the technique.

ADVANTAGES AND DISADVANTAGES

Before listing the supposed advantages of the bisecting technique, it should again be stated that the consensus of opinion now is that the paralleling technique is the technique of choice for periapical radiography.[1]

Advantages

The bisecting-angle technique is said to be easier to perform and is still used by many dentists in practice at this time. The use of the patient's finger or simple bite blocks for holding the film packets in position avoids the use of the bulky paralleling instruments. In patients with small mouths, children, and patients with low palatal vaults, paralleling devices may be extremely difficult to use.

Since the film is held close to the tooth, it is possible to use an 8-inch FFD, and the objectional, "bulky," extension cylinder necessary in the paralleling technique can be avoided. This objection is not valid in the newer machines with the extended FFD within the tube head.

Shorter exposure times can be used in the bisecting technique because of the shorter FFD; hence there is less chance for patient movement. In reality, this may not be a valid objection. With the use of faster film we are comparing exposure times of $^1/_{10}$ vs $^4/_{10}$ second (inverse square law). Previously, with the use of slower films, the possibility of movement with a 4-second exposure compared to a 1-second exposure was greater, and the advantage had greater validity.

Disadvantages

The major disadvantage of the bisecting technique is that the image projected on the film is dimensionally distorted (see Chapter 3).

The bisecting technique is difficult to perform with the patient in a contour chair in the supine position as utilized in four-handed dentistry. It is very hard to place the patient in this position so that the occlusal plane of the jaw being radiographed is parallel to the floor. All vertical angulations used in the bisecting technique are measured from this line.

Other disadvantages of the bisecting technique are related to the use of an 8-inch FFD. The 8-inch FFD when compared to the extended 16-inch FFD causes greater image enlargement and distortion (see Fig. 1-27). There is also more tissue volume exposed with an 8-inch FFD than with a 16-inch FFD (see Chapter 2).

METHOD

In this periapical technique, the film is held as close to the tooth as possible, without bending the film. The long axis of the film will therefore not be parallel to the long axis of the tooth. An imaginary line is drawn to bisect the angle formed by the long axis of the tooth and the plane of the film. The central ray of the x-ray beam is directed perpendicular to this bisecting line; this determines the vertical angulation of the x-ray beam (see Fig. 1-30). For the maxillary teeth, positive angulations (PID pointing down) are used, and for mandibular teeth, negative angulations (PID pointing up) are used. At 0-degree angulations, the PID is parallel to the floor; this becomes the reference point from which vertical angulations are measured. Therefore, it is important to have the occlusal plane of the jaw being radiographed positioned parallel to the floor.

THE FULL-MOUTH SERIES

Maxillary central and lateral incisors (left or right) (Fig. 4-1)

Chair position. The maxillary occlusal plane is positioned parallel to the floor, and the sagittal plane of the patient's face is perpendicular to the floor.

Film position. The film packet is held vertically so that it extends evenly ⅛ inch below the incisal edge of the incisors. The midpoint of this ⅛-inch border should be between the lateral and central incisors. The film packet is held as close to the lingual surface of the incisors as possible without bending it. The film packet is held in position by the patient's thumb of the opposite hand.

Point of entry. The central ray is directed just below the midpoint of the nares, aimed at the center of the film packet.

Vertical angulation. $+50°$.

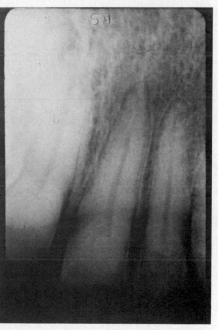

Fig. 4-1. Maxillary central and lateral incisors. **A,** Film packet and PID. Dot represents point of entry. **B,** Radiograph. **C,** Diagram.

B

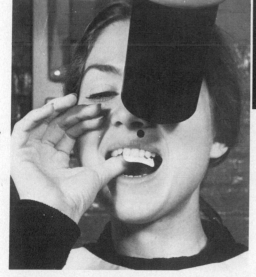

A

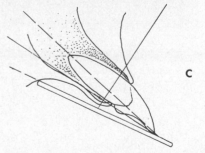

C

Horizontal angulation. The central ray is perpendicular to the film packet in the horizontal plane.

If only one film is to be used for the right and left maxillary central and lateral incisors, the center of the film packet is placed between the central incisors, and the central ray is directed just below the tip of the nose (Fig. 4-2).

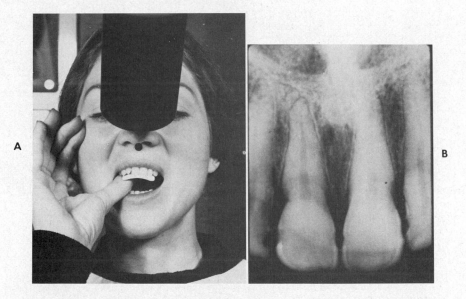

A   B

Fig. 4-2. Right and left central and lateral incisors. **A,** Film packet and PID. Dot represents point of entry. **B,** Radiograph.

Maxillary canines (Fig. 4-3)

Chair position. The maxillary occlusal plane is positioned parallel to the floor, and the sagittal plane of the patient's face is perpendicular to the floor.

Film position. The film packet is held vertically and extends ⅛ inch below the tip of the canine. The canine is in the center of the film packet, which is held firmly against the lingual surface of the canine with the patient's thumb of the opposite hand.

Point of entry. The central ray is directed at the base of the lateral nasal grove, aimed at the center of the film packet.

Vertical angulation. +50°.

Horizontal angulation. The central ray is perpendicular to the film packet in the horizontal plane.

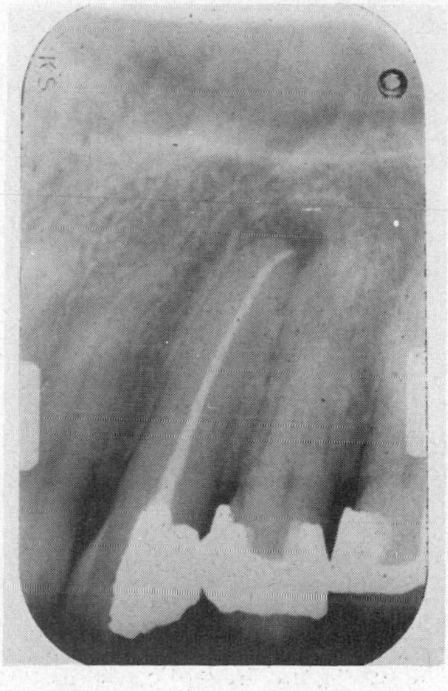

Fig. 4-3. Maxillary canine. **A,** Film packet and PID. **B,** Radiograph. **C,** Diagram.

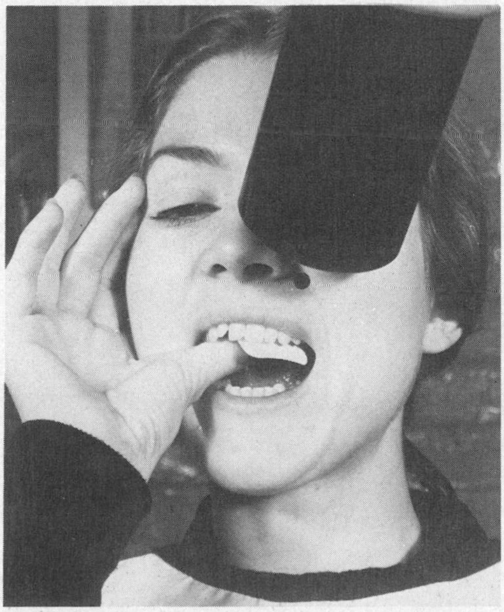

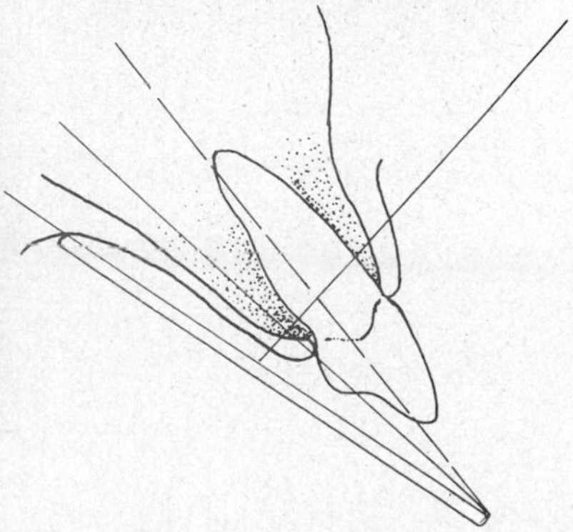

Maxillary premolars (Fig. 4-4)

Chair position. The maxillary occlusal plane is positioned parallel to the floor and the sagittal plane of the patient's face is perpendicular to the floor.

Film position. The film packet is held horizontally and extends ⅛ inch below the occlusal surfaces of the teeth. The second premolar is in the center of the film packet. The packet is held in position against the lingual surfaces by the patient's thumb of the opposite hand. The operator should avoid shaping the packet to the arch.

Point of entry. The central ray is directed at the most anterior part of the cheek-bone, aimed at the center of the film packet.

Vertical angulation. +40°.

Horizontal angulation. The central ray is perpendicular to the film packet in the horizontal plane and is directed through the interproximal spaces.

Fig. 4-4. Maxillary premolars. **A,** Film packet and PID. **B,** Radiograph. **C,** Diagram.

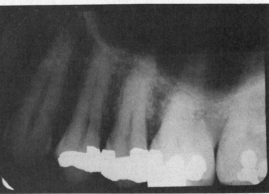

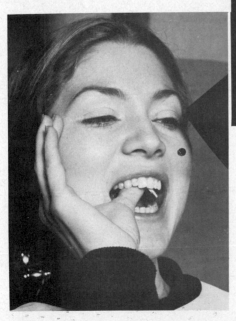

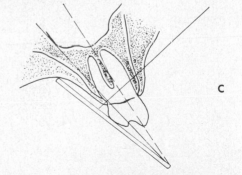

A

B

C

Maxillary molars (Fig. 4-5)

Chair position. The maxillary occlusal plane is positioned parallel to the floor, and the sagittal plane of the patient's face is perpendicular to the floor.

Film position. The film is held horizontally and extends ⅛ inch evenly below the occlusal surfaces of the teeth. The second molar is in the center of the film packet. The film packet is held against the lingual surfaces of the teeth by the patient's thumb of the opposite hand.

Point of entry. The central ray is directed through the zygomatic arch at the center of the film. The distal curvature of the open-ended cone should not be distal to the outer canthus (corner) of the eye.

Vertical angulation. $+30°$.

Horizontal angulation. The central ray is perpendicular to the film packet in the horizontal plane and is directed through the interproximal spaces.

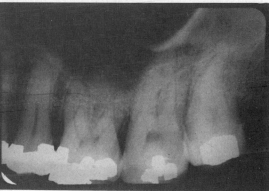

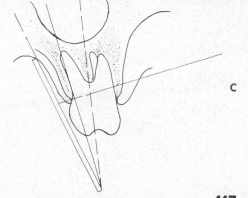

Fig. 4-5. Maxillary molars. **A,** Film packet and PID. **B,** Radiograph. **C,** Diagram.

B

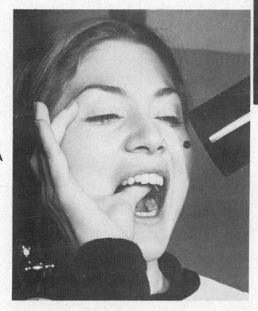

A

C

117

BITE-WING PROJECTIONS (see Chapter 3)

Mandibular incisors (Fig. 4-6)

Chair position. The patient is positioned so that when the mouth is open the mandibular occlusal plane is parallel to the floor, and the sagittal plane of the patient's face is perpendicular to the floor.

Film position. The film is held vertically so that it extends ⅛ inch above the incisal edges of the incisors. The midpoint of this ⅛-inch border should be between the central incisors. All four lower incisors will be seen on one film. The film is held against the lingual surfaces of the incisors by the patient's index finger.

Point of entry. The central ray is directed at the depression in the face just above the chin (mental groove), aimed at the center of the film.

Vertical angulation. $-20°$.

Horizontal angulation. The central ray is perpendicular to the film in the horizontal plane.

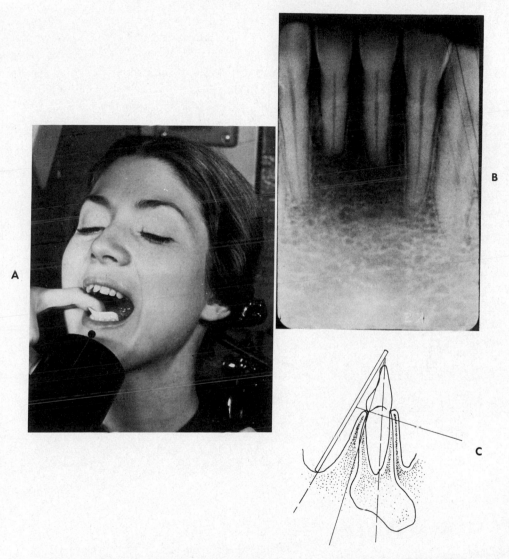

Fig. 4-6. Mandibular incisors. **A,** Film packet and PID. **B,** Radiograph. **C,** Diagram.

119

Mandibular canines (Fig. 4-7)

Chair position. The patient is positioned so that when the mouth is open the mandibular occlusal plane is parallel to the floor, and the sagittal plane of the patient's face is perpendicular to the floor.

Film position. The film packet is held vertically and extends ⅛ inch above the tip of the canine, which is in the center of the film packet. The film packet is held against the lingual surface of the canine with the index finger of the patient's opposite hand.

Point of entry. The central ray is directed at the root of the canine, aimed at the middle of the film packet.

Vertical angulation. −20°.

Horizontal angulation. The central ray is perpendicular to the film in the horizontal plane.

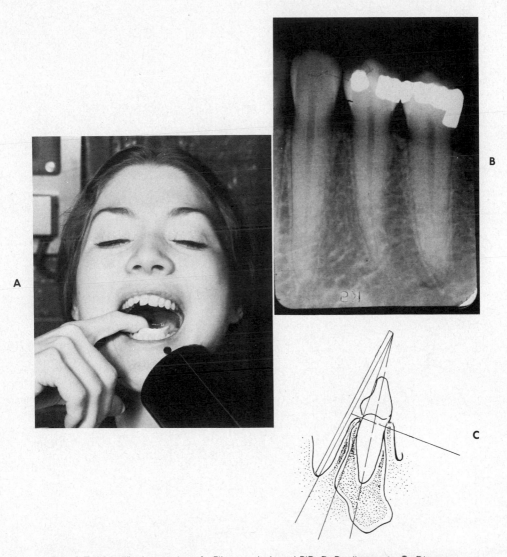

Fig. 4-7. Mandibular canine. **A,** Film packet and PID. **B,** Radiograph. **C,** Diagram.

Mandibular premolars (Fig. 4-8)

Chair position. The patient is positioned so that when the mouth is open the mandibular occlusal plane is parallel to the floor, and the sagittal plane of the patient's face is perpendicular to the floor.

Film position. The film packet is held horizontally and extends ⅛ inch above the occlusal surfaces of the teeth. The second premolar is in the center of the film. The film packet is held against the lingual surfaces of the teeth by the index finger of the patient's opposite hand.

Point of entry. The central ray is directed at the mental foramen, aimed at the center of the film packet.

Vertical angulation. −15°.

Horizontal angulation. The central ray is perpendicular to the film in the horizontal plane.

Fig. 4-8. Mandibular premolars. **A,** Film packet and PID. **B,** Radiograph. **C,** Diagram.

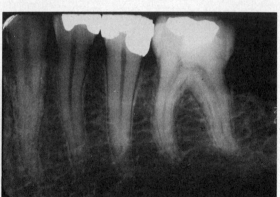

B

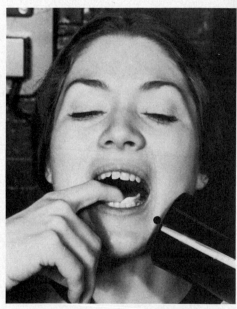

A

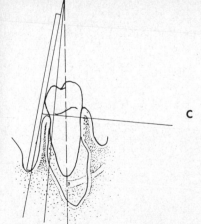

C

Mandibular molars (Fig. 4-9)

Chair position. The patient is positioned so that when the mouth is open the mandibular occlusal plane is parallel to the floor, and the sagittal plane of the patient's face is perpendicular to the floor.

Film position. The film packet is held horizontally and extends ⅛ inch above the occlusal surfaces of the molars. The second molar is in the middle of the film. The film is held agsinst the lingual surface of the molars by the index finger of the patient's opposite hand. Because of the anatomy of the area the film packet will almost be parallel to the long axis of the tooth.

Point of entry. The central ray is directed at the roots of the molars, aimed at the center of the film packet.

Vertical angulation. −5°.

Horizontal angulation. The central ray is directed perpendicular to the film packet in the horizontal plane.

Fig. 4-9. Mandibular molars. **A,** Film packet and PID. **B,** Radiograph. **C,** Diagram.

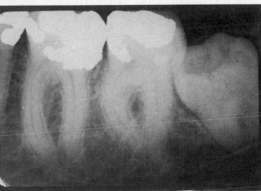

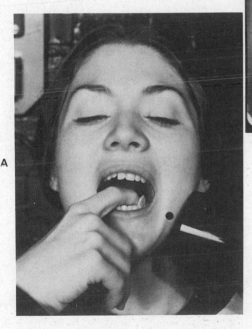

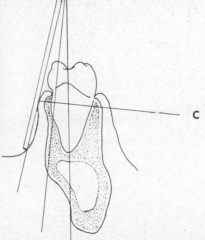

A

B

C

123

COMMON ERRORS

The following are the most common errors seen in the bisecting technique. Recognition and correction of occasional errors in technique are important. Not all patients are cooperative or have anatomically large mouths that are easy to radiograph. It should be remembered that films retaken because of poor technique add unnecessarily to the patient's radiation burden (see Chapter 3 for other chairside errors).

Elongation (Fig. 4-10)

Elongation, or lengthening of the image on the film, can be caused by too little vertical angulation, improper occlusal plane orientation because of patient position, or poor film placement.

Remedy. Make sure the film and the central ray are in the correct relationship. In the bisecting-angle technique the vertical angulation should be increased to correct elongation. The occlusal plane of the jaw being radiographed should be parallel to the floor. Patients tend to move after a few exposures, or lift their heads to watch the operator. Their movements disorient the occlusal plane. Check the patient's head position before making each exposure.

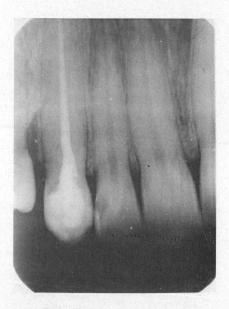

Fig. 4-10. Elongated image.

Foreshortening (Fig. 4-11)

Foreshortening, the shortening of the image on the film, is not as frequent an error as elongation. It can be caused by excessive vertical angulation or poor occlusal plane orientation.

Remedy. In the bisecting-angle technique decrease the vertical angulation to overcome errors of foreshortening.

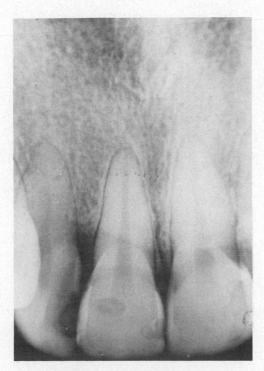

Fig. 4-11. Foreshortened image.

Sagittal plane orientation (Fig. 4-12)

When periapical radiographs show the occlusal surfaces of the teeth, the patient's head has tipped away from the proper sagittal plane. This will be accompanied by elongation of the image.

Remedy. Make sure the patient does not tip his head away from the tube head as it is brought into approximation with the skin.

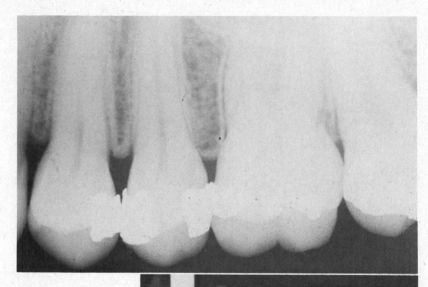

A

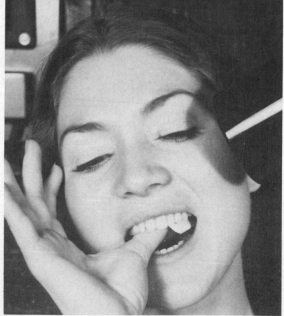

B

Fig. 4-12. A, Elongated and distorted radiograph caused by poor sagittal plane orientation of patient's head. **B,** Poor sagittal plane orientation.

EDENTULOUS SERIES

A full-mouth series of radiographs is taken even though the patient may be wholly or partially edentulous. The fact that there are no teeth present in an area of the mouth does not preclude the possibility of retained roots, impacted teeth, cysts, and other pathologic conditions present in the bone. The edentulous series is composed of 13 periapical films. The bite-wing films are not taken, since there are no teeth to support the tabs, and only one film is used in the maxillary central, lateral, and canine area (Fig. 4-13). In small edentulous mouths an 11 film survey may suffice by using only one mandibular anterior periapical film and extending the premolar projection anteriorly to include the canine area.

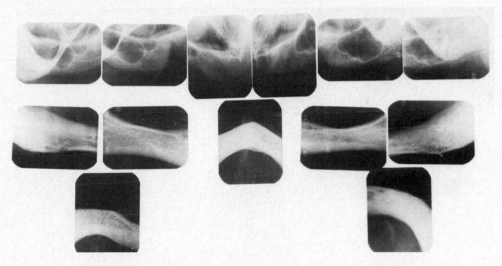

Fig. 4-13. A 13-film edentulous survey.

The films are positioned in the same way as a regular series but with certain modifications. The crest of the edentulous ridge replaces the occlusal plane of the teeth as the plane of orientation. The film is positioned either ⅛ inch above or below the ridge. Since there are no teeth and there may be a great deal of ridge resorption, the film will lie flatter against the palate or in the floor of the mouth, increasing the angle to be bisected. The vertical angulation will then have to be much greater. The best guideline in the edentulous series is to adjust the vertical angulation so that the central ray is almost perpendicular to the film. Any slight foreshortening that may result will not affect the diagnosis of any intrabony conditions. If the paralleling technique is used, extra cotton rolls may be necessary to support the holding device while the film is kept parallel to the edentulous ridge.

The exposure times are reduced by a factor of one fourth for the edentulous series.

There are two possible alternatives to the edentulous periapical survey. The first is a panoramic survey (Fig. 4-14). The second and more universal method would be the use of topographic occlusal film projections. The entire maxillary and mandibular ridge can usually be seen in their respective occlusal projections (Fig. 4-15). These are survey films and if any suspicious areas are seen, a periapical projection of the area is done to make a definitive diagnosis.

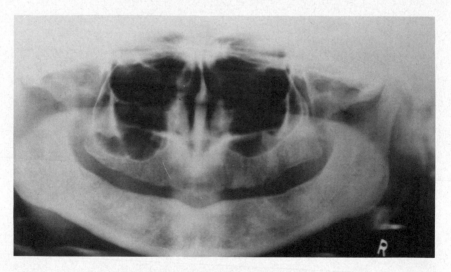

Fig. 4-14. Edentulous panoramic survey.

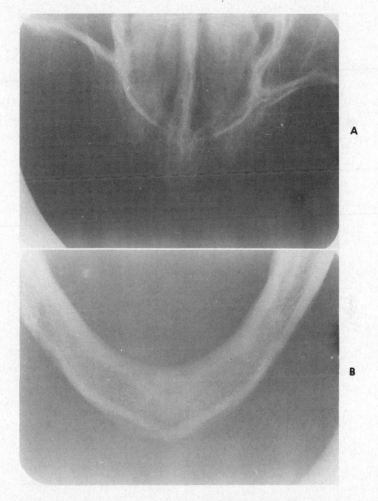

Fig. 4-15. A, Edentulous occlusal survey of maxilla. **B,** Edentulous occlusal survey of mandible.

PEDODONTIC FULL-MOUTH SERIES

Depending on the age of the child, the composition of the full-mouth series may vary. The size of the child's mouth is the determining factor.

Up to the age of 5 it is necessary to use the pedodontic size film ($\frac{7}{8} \times 1\frac{3}{8}$ inches) for anterior, posterior, and bite-wing projections. The full-mouth series at this age will be 12 films: three maxillary anterior films, three mandibular anterior films, four mandibular and maxillary premolar-molar projections, and two bite-wing projections. The size of the child's mouth does not necessitate separate premolar and molar films. For the same reason, only one bite-wing film is taken on each side.

In the 6- to 9-year old group the pedodontic film or narrow adult film ($\frac{15}{16} \times 1\frac{9}{16}$ inches) can be used for anterior projections since the child's arch shape at this age can still be very narrow. For the posterior projections adult size ($1\frac{1}{4} \times 1\frac{5}{8}$ inches), narrow adult, or pedodontic film is used depending on the size of the arch. At this age two posterior periapical films are taken since the 6-year molars have erupted and the dental arch has lengthened. One bite-wing film on each side is also used.

After age 9 the full adult series is taken, using the narrow adult film where necessary. These age guidelines are flexible depending on the growth and development of the child. As a rule it is best to use the largest film size that can be comfortably accommodated by the patient (Fig. 4-16).

In the pedodontic series the chair position, film placement, point of entry, and vertical and horizontal angulations follow the same rules as in the adult series in both the bisecting-angle and the paralleling techniques.

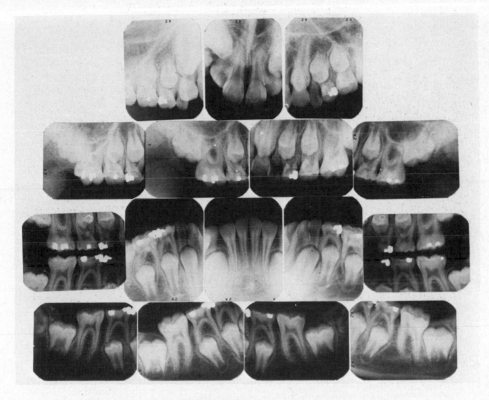

Fig. 4-16. Full-mouth pedodontic survey of a 9-year-old patient.

STUDY QUESTIONS

1. What is the proper chair position for radiography using the bisecting-angle technique?
2. Explain the theory of the bisecting-angle technique.
3. What are the advantages and disadvantages of this technique?
4. What do the terms point of entry, vertical angulation, and horizontal angulation mean?
5. Why is a full-mouth series of radiographs necessary for an edentulous patient?
6. What causes elongated and foreshortened images on radiographs?
7. What causes overlapping of images on radiographs?
8. What is the correct sagittal plane orientation for the patient's head? What errors are caused by poor orientation?
9. What determines the variations in degree of vertical angulation from projection to projection in the bisecting-angle technique?
10. What are two possible alternatives to a 13-film edentulous survey?

REFERENCE

1. A summary of recommendations from the technology assessment forum, National Center for Health Care Technology, J. Am. Dent. Assoc. **103**:423-425, September 1981.

chapter 5   Accessory radiographic techniques

Dental radiography does not limit itself to the intraoral periapical and bite-wing films that have been previously described. There are many accessory techniques, intraoral and extraoral, using different sizes of film, different projections, and other types of x-ray machines such as the panoramic units. Most of the accessory techniques can be performed with the conventional dental x-ray unit.

As with intraoral radiography, the dental auxiliary should be knowledgeable and skilled in these accessory techniques. However, some states have laws that prohibit the dental auxiliary from performing certain extraoral techniques. Information about these restrictions is readily available from the appropriate agencies in the individual states.

OCCLUSAL FILM PROJECTIONS

Occlusal film projections are used to localize objects and pathologic conditions in the buccolingual dimension and to visualize areas that would not be seen on periapical films because of the insufficient field size. A right-angle occlusal technique is used, for localizing in the buccolingual dimension; the topographic occlusal technique is used for the large pathologic areas.

Right-angle projections

In right-angle projections the central ray is directed at an angle of 90 degrees to the film. For example, this technique would be used to locate an object such as an impacted tooth in the third dimension. We have mentioned previously that dental radiographs picture a three-dimensional subject in a two-dimensional plane, usually vertical and horizontal. The radiographs do not indicate depth. In the example of the impacted tooth, we might know from a conventional radiograph its mesiodistal location and its vertical height from the crest of the alveolar ridge, but we would not know its depth in the bone in a buccolingual dimension. One way to determine whether an impacted mandibular molar lies buccal or lingual to the alveolar ridge is to take a radiograph from another direction. In this example it would be an occlusal radiograph with the central ray coming from underneath the mandible, directed at a right angle to a film placed on the occlusal surface of the mandibular teeth.

Topographic projections

The angulation of the topographic projection may vary from 45 to 75 degrees depending on the anatomic area. Since the occlusal packet is approximately 4 times the size of the intraoral packet, it can record areas that would not be seen on the smaller film. The extreme vertical angulations are necessary to compensate for the lack of parallelism between the object and the film. This is a modification of the bisecting-angle technique.

Packet

The occlusal film packet is 2¼ × 3 inches and is supplied in either single or double films (Fig. 5-1). These films are sometimes called "sandwich films" because they are positioned in the patient's mouth with the teeth closed on the film packet, resembling the biting of a sandwich. Occlusal films are processed in the darkroom in the same way as other intraoral films.

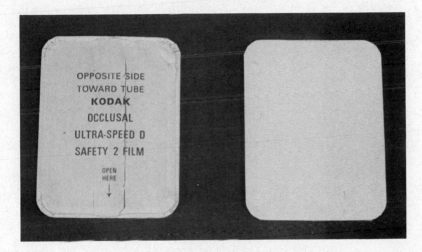

OPPOSITE SIDE
TOWARD TUBE
KODAK
OCCLUSAL
ULTRA-SPEED D
SAFETY 2 FILM

OPEN
HERE
↓

Fig. 5-1. Front and back of occlusal film packet.

Mandibular occlusal technique

In the mandibular occlusal technique the film packet is placed in the patient's mouth on the occlusal surfaces of the lower teeth. The back of the film packet faces the palate, with the front of the packet facing the tongue on the occlusal surfaces of the lower teeth. In patients with small mouths it will be possible to get both right and left sides of the mandible on one film if it is inserted with the longer side extending across the patient's mouth. In patients with larger mouths it may be necessary to take separate film of each half of the mandible. In this instance the longest dimension of the film packet

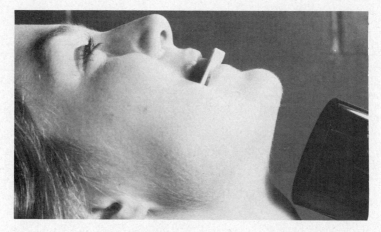

Fig. 5-2. Film placement and cone position for mandibular occlusal film. Note that central ray is directed at 90 degrees to center of film packet.

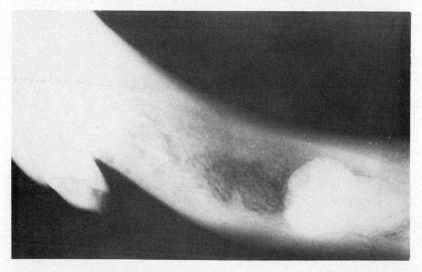

Fig. 5-3. Occlusal radiograph of patient's mandibular posterior area. Note buccal and lingual cortex of bone and impacted molar.

will run anteroposteriorly. The film is placed as far posterior on the mandible as possible so that the edge of the packet touches the ascending ramus of the mandible. The patient is directed to bite gently on the film packet. For the right-angle projection the central ray of the x-ray beam is directed from under the mandible so that it is perpendicular to the center of the film packet (Figs. 5-2 and 5-3). For the topographic view of the mandible, the central ray is directed at a point just above the mental eminence at a vertical angulation of 65 degrees. To accomplish these angulations it is necessary for the operator to tip the headrest of the chair back and have the patient extend his head and neck posteriorly (Figs. 5-4 and 5-5).

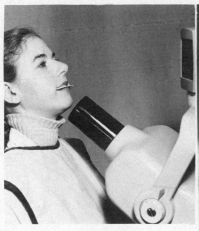

Fig. 5-4

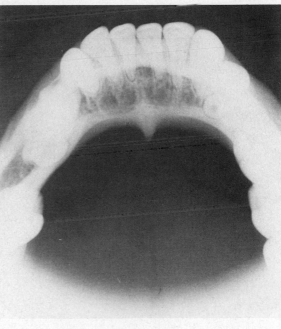

Fig. 5-4. Topographic mandibular occlusal projection.
Fig. 5-5. Topographic occlusal projection of mandible.

Fig. 5-5

Maxillary occlusal technique

In an anterior topographic occlusal view of the maxilla, the film packet is placed in the patient's mouth with the front of the film packet facing the palate and the long dimension of the packet running across the mouth. The packet is positioned as far posterior as possible so that the posterior edge of the film packet touches the ascending ramus of the mandible. With the patient's head positioned so that the film plane is parallel to the floor, the central ray is directed at a 65-degree vertical angulation through the bridge of the nose (Figs. 5-6 and 5-7). In the right-angle occlusal view of the maxilla, the film is placed in the same position in the patient's mouth, but the central ray is directed perpendicular to the center of the film packet. To do this the PID must be positioned above the head of the patient at about the hairline. The vertical angulation is 90 degrees. Since there is an increased FFD when compared with the maxillary topographic view, this projection will require a longer exposure time (Figs. 5-8 and 5-9).

The posterior topographic view can be considered a topographic view of the maxillary sinus. The film packet is positioned either on the left or the right side of the patient's mouth, from the midline, laterally with the long side running anteroposteriorly. The central ray is directed to a point just above the apices of the premolars at a vertical angulation of 55 degrees (Figs. 5-10 and 5-11).

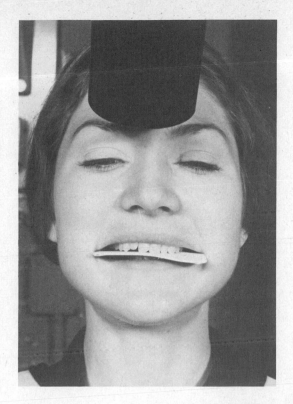

Fig. 5-6. Film placement and cone position for topographic occlusal view of maxilla. Note that central ray is directed at 65 degrees to bridge of nose.

Fig. 5-7. Occlusal radiograph of the maxilla, topographic view.

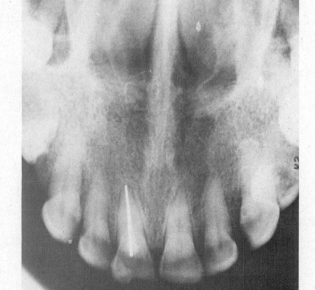

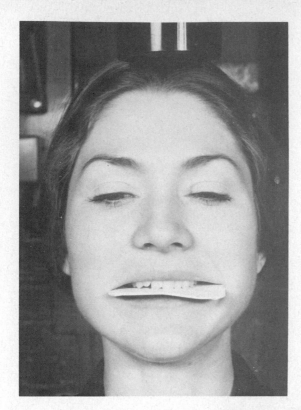

Fig. 5-8. Film placement and cone position for a true occlusal view of maxilla. Note that central ray is directed at 90 degrees to film packet.

Fig. 5-9. Right angle occlusal projection of maxilla showing palatal relationship of impacted canine.

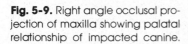

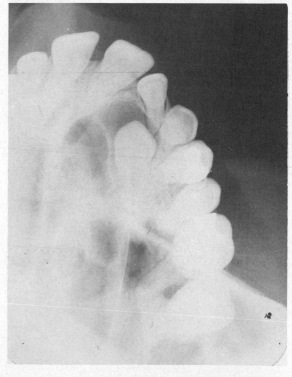

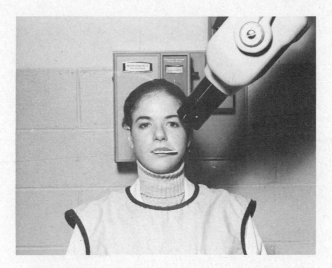

Fig. 5-10. Posterior topographic occlusal projection.

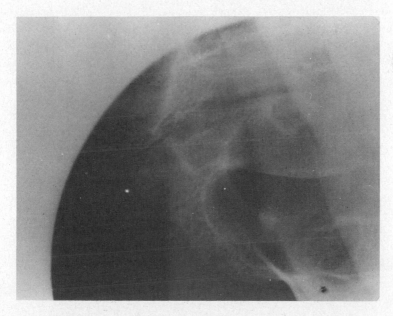

Fig. 5-11. Topographic occlusal radiograph of maxillary sinus.

EXTRAORAL PROJECTIONS

Indications

There are two indications for the use of extraoral radiographs. The first is a situation where a patient cannot or will not open his mouth to allow the film packet to be placed intraorally. Uncooperative or handicapped patients may refuse or be unable to open their mouths for film placement. Patients with trismus as well as patients with temporomandibular joint ankylosis will be unable to open their mouths.

The second indication is when the area being radiographed is larger than or cannot be seen on intraoral films. There are many areas of the mandible and maxilla that cannot be seen on intraoral films. The scope of dental treatment is not limited to the teeth and alveolar bone. It may be necessary to radiograph such areas as the angle and ramus of the mandible, the temporomandibular joint, maxillary sinus, or lesions that grow so large that they cannot be completely seen on periapical films.

Equipment

The equipment needed to do standard extraoral projections is minimal and not too costly. Extraoral techniques require a regular dental x-ray unit, film cassette, 8- × 10- or 5- × 7-inch, film, intensifying screens, and cassette holders or angling boards.

X-ray unit. Extraoral radiographs can be taken with a standard dental x-ray unit. The x-ray machine must be positioned so that a minimum FFD of 36 inches can be achieved. This is necessary to get a sufficiently large beam size at the patient's face.

Films. Extraoral film may vary in size, but the most common sizes used are 5 × 7 or 8 × 10 inches. Two types of film are available: one for use with intensifying screens and the other for use without screens. The screen film is more sensitive to the light emitted by the intensifying screens than it is to radiation. These films should not be interchanged; that is, nonscreen film should not be used with intensifying screens or screen films used without intensifying screens.

The sheets of extraoral film come individually wrapped in boxes of 25 or 50. A common mistake is to place the extraoral film in the cassette without removing the film's paper cover. The paper blocks the light emitted by the intensifying screen during the exposure and negates the action of the screen, leading to an underexposed film.

Cassettes. The films are contained in a carrier called a cassette. The cassette can be rigid or flexible and can come in varying sizes corresponding to the size of the film used (Fig. 5-12). The rigid cassette may be cardboard, metal, plastic, or a combination of these. A cassette must be light-tight and yet allow the passage of x-rays to affect the x-ray film contained within the cassette. The film packet wrapping in intraoral film could also be considered a cassette—a paper cassette—although it is never referred to as such.

Cassettes must be marked with lead letters to identify whether the film is of the left or right, or it will not be possible to orient the finished radiograph. Extraoral films have no raised dot to signify which side of the film should face the x-ray tube. Lead strips are also available that will imprint the patient's name and the date on the film.

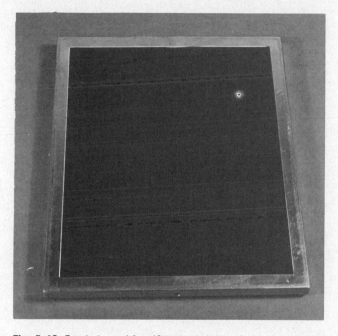

Fig. 5-12. Front view of 8 × 10 inch metal-and-plastic cassette.

Intensifying screens. Metal and plastic cassettes usually contain intensifying screens (Fig. 5-13). As the name implies, these screens intensify or increase the radiation and thus decrease the exposure time. This happens because the screens are usually coated with calcium tungstate, a substance that has the property of fluorescence. Such a substance will emit light when struck by x radiation. In the film cassette the light emitted is in the same pattern as the x-rays that have penetrated the object, so the film inside the cassette is affected by both x-rays and light. However, there is a loss of image detail with this intensification of the x-ray beam. An extraoral film can never give image detail equal to that obtained with intraoral films (Fig. 5-14).

Intensifying screens vary in their speed or exposure time requirements, just as film does. As in film, the size of the crystals that make up the screen determine the speed of the screen. The larger the calcium tungstate crystals, the faster the screen, but the poorer the definition. In dentistry we usually use fast screens for extraoral work because the lesions we are looking for are marked by gross changes. An extraoral projection using intensifying screens would not be the procedure of choice when looking for recurrent decay or a thickened periodontal membrane.

When cassettes are loaded or unloaded in the darkroom, care should be taken to not scratch the intensifying screens with sharp objects such as film racks. If an intensifying screen is badly scratched and the calcium tungstate completely removed, a white streak will appear on the film taken with this screen.

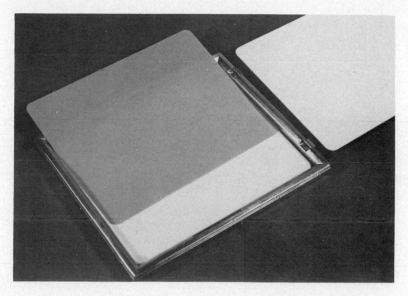

Fig. 5-13. Cassette in open position, showing front and back intensifying screens and piece of film.

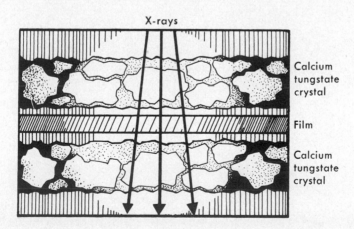

Fig. 5-14. Diagram of effect of x-rays on intensifying screens. Note halo of light produced at periphery that reduces radiographic definition.

Holding devices. Extraoral film holders are available that can be wall mounted or used on a tabletop. If no device is available, the patient can hold the cassette. Holding devices have the advantage of standardizing techniques and preventing patient and film movement (Fig. 5-15).

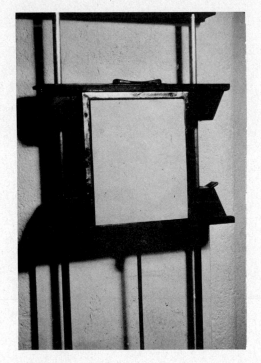

Fig. 5-15. Cassette in wall-mounted film-holding device.

Film sensitivity and processing

Extraoral screen films are more sensitive to light than are intraoral films. Therefore, what would be acceptable safelight conditions in the darkroom for processing intraoral films might fog the extraoral films. The films used in panoramic radiography are especially sensitive to excessive safelighting and may be not merely fogged but entirely ruined. Safelighting should always be checked before processing extraoral films.

Extraoral films are processed in the same manner as intraoral films. The time-temperature method is used with the same fixation and washing time as with intraoral films. The only difference is that special sizes of film hangers are used. Special care should be taken when processing the large films, because they are easier to scratch when more than one film is being processed at a time (Fig. 5-16).

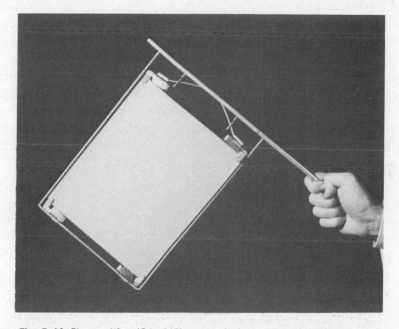

Fig. 5-16. Piece of 8 × 10 inch film mounted on a processing film hanger.

Projections

As in intraoral radiography there are certain factors that must be known for every projection made. These factors are: (1) the relationship of the film to the patient, (2) the relationship of the central ray of the x-ray beam to the patient and the film, (3) the FFD, (4) the point of entry of the x-ray beam, (5) the kVp, and (6) the mAs.

Suggested exposure times and mA and kVp settings are given but these may vary depending on the speed of the film and intensifying screen used as well as the size of the patient.

Lateral oblique projection of the mandible. The lateral oblique projection of the mandible is used for surveying one side of the mandible from the distal of the canine to the angle, ramus, condyle, and coronoid process. It is not diagnostic anterior to the canine because of the superimposition caused by the anterior curve of the mandible. Before the advent of panoramic techniques, it was the most often used extraoral technique because it is ideal for showing mandibular third molar impactions as well as other mandibular pathologic conditions.

An 8- × 10-inch or 5- × 7-inch cassette may be used for this projection. The cassette is supported by the patient's shoulder or a holding device on the side of the mandible to be radiographed. The cassette is in contact with the cheekbone and mandible. The patient's head is inclined about 15 degrees away from the x-ray tube. The central ray is directed from under the opposite side of the mandible at right angles to the cassette. The FFD is 14 inches. An average exposure time at 65 kVp and 10 mA using fast film and screens would be 20 impulses ($\frac{1}{3}$ second) (Fig. 5-17).

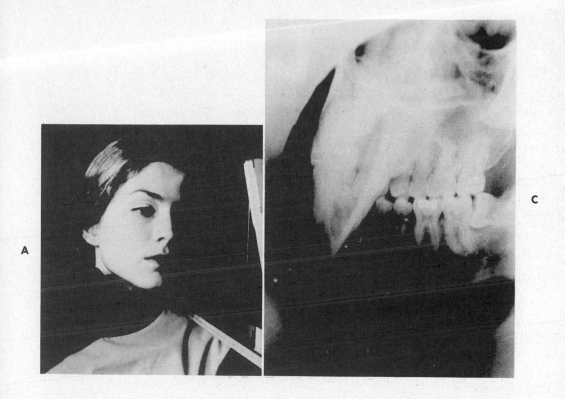

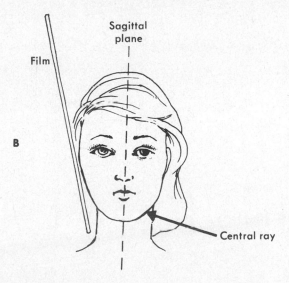

Fig. 5-17. Lateral oblique projection. **A,** Central ray is directed at cassette from beneath opposite side of mandible. **B,** Drawing. **C,** Radiograph.

149

Lateral skull projection. The lateral skull projection is used to survey the whole skull. The right and left sides of the skull are superimposed upon each other, with the side nearer the tube magnified slightly more than the side nearer the film. It is used in dentistry to detect fractures and systemic pathologic conditions such as Paget's disease and is the projection used in lateral cephalometric measurement in orthodontics.

An 8- × 10-inch cassette is used, usually with intensifying screens. The cassette is held in position by the patient, supported on the patient's shoulder or by some supportive device. The cassette is positioned parallel to the sagittal plane of the skull. The central ray is directed at the external auditory meatus at an FFD of 36 inches. The vertical angulation is 0 degrees. An average exposure time for an adult, using fast film and screens at 65 kVp and 10 mA, would be 30 impulses (½ second) (Fig. 5-18).

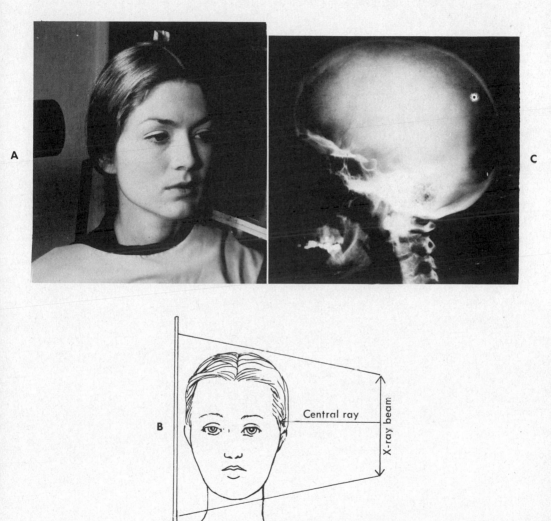

Fig. 5-18. Lateral skull projection. **A,** Central ray is directed at external auditory meatus at a minimum FFD of 36 inches. **B,** Drawing. **C,** Radiograph.

Posteroanterior projection. The posteroanterior projection is used to survey the skull in the anteroposterior plane and provides a means of localizing changes in a mediolateral direction. The left and right sides of the facial structures are not superimposed upon each other as in the lateral skull projection. In dentistry this projection is used to detect fractures and their displacements, tumors, and large areas of disease. It is not effective for studying the maxillary sinus because of the superimposition of other cranial structures.

An 8- × 10-inch cassette is used, usually with intensifying screens. The cassette can be held in position by the patient, but some type of cassette-holding device is preferable. The patient is positioned with his nose and forehead touching the cassette. The central ray is directed at a 0-degree vertical angulation, aimed at the external occipital protuberance (the prominent bump near the base of the skull). The FFD is 36 inches. An average exposure time using fast film and screens at 65 kVp and 10 mA would be 30 impulses (½ second) (Fig. 5-19).

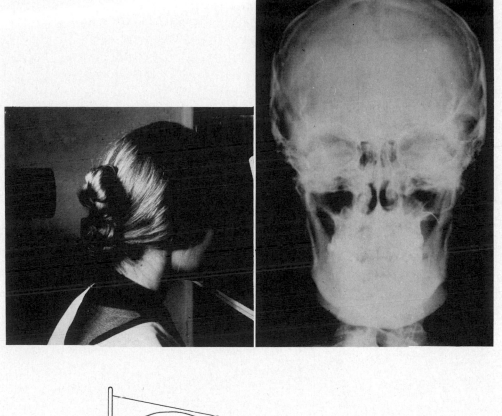

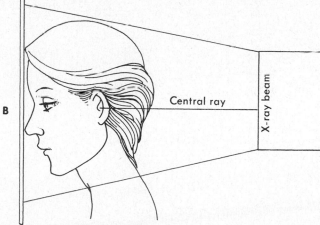

Fig. 5-19. Posteroanterior projection. **A,** Central ray directed at occipital protuberance at minimum FFD of 36 inches. **B,** Drawing. **C,** Radiograph.

Posteroanterior (Waters') view of the sinuses. Waters' view is a variation of the posteroanterior projection that enlarges the middle third of the face and is useful in diagnoses of maxillary sinus and other pathologic conditions occurring in the middle third of the face. It differs from the posteroanterior projection positioning in that the patient's mouth is kept open while his nose and chin are touching the cassette. The central ray is again directed at the external occipital protuberance and an FFD of 36 inches is used. An average exposure time at 65 kVp and 10 mA would be 45 impulses (¾ second) (Fig. 5-20).

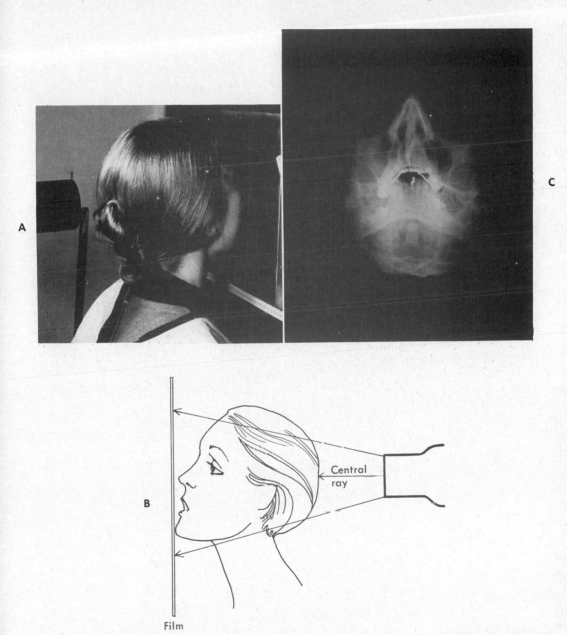

Fig. 5-20. Posteroanterior projection of the sinuses (Waters' view). **A,** Central ray is directed perpendicular to cassette at occipital protuberance using 36-inch FFD. **B,** Drawing. **C,** Radiograph.

155

Temporomandibular joint, transcranial projection. The temporomandibular joint is difficult to radiograph well because of its anatomic location. It is bordered medially by the petrous portion of the temporal bone and laterally by the zygomatic arch. Yet it is necessary to examine the condyle to look for such conditions as calcifications, ankylosis, arthritis changes, fractures, and tumors. The transcranial technique positions the cassette and the central ray so as to avoid the superimposition of these structures.

A 5- × 7-inch cassette can be used if only one exposure is going to be made. Usually radiographs are taken of both the left and right condyles in both the open and closed positions. Since the diagnostic area is relatively small, the four views can be placed on a 8- × 10-inch film if appropriate lead shielding is used on the cassette. The patient's head is positioned parallel to the cassette with the side to be radiographed closest to the cassette. The cassette can be supported on the patient's shoulder or on a positioning device. The point of entry for the central ray of the x-ray beam is on the opposite side of the head from the condyle being radiographed, approximately 2½ inches above and ½ inch in front of the external auditory meatus. The x-ray beam is directed at a vertical angulation of 25 to 30 degrees. The end of the PID approximates the skin. An average exposure time at 65 kVp and 10 mA using fast film and screens would be 30 impulses (½ second) (Fig. 5-21).

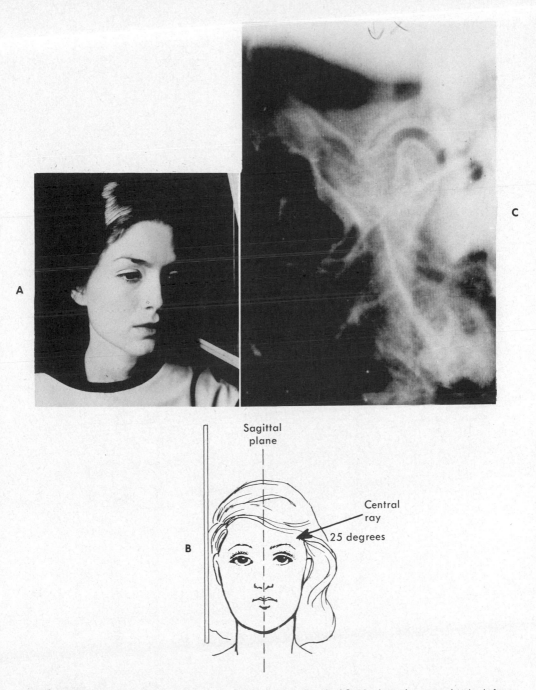

Fig. 5-21. Transcranial TMJ projection. **A,** Central ray is directed 2½ inches above and ½ inch forward of external auditory meatus with vertical angulation of 25-30 degrees. **B,** Drawing. **C,** Radiograph.

157

There are available temporomandibular joint positioning boards that are based on the transcranial technique that also incorporate means to hold the patient in a fixed position while allowing for movement of the cassette to give up to three exposures for each condyle (open, closed, and at rest) on a 8- × 10-inch film (Fig. 5-22).

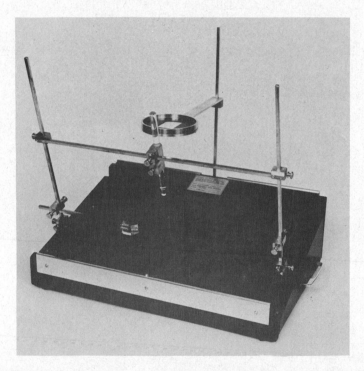

Fig. 5-22. TMJ angling board. (Courtesy Margraf Dental Mfg. Inc., Jenkintown, Pa.)

PANORAMIC RADIOGRAPHY

Panoramic radiography refers to a technique that will produce a film that shows the patient's upper and lower jaws on one film. There are two techniques that are currently being used to produce these films. The first is the use of an intraoral x-ray source where the tube is placed in the patient's mouth and the film wrapped externally around the patient's face. This technique is not commonly used, and the radiographs produced show a great deal of distortion but the radiation exposure is significantly decreased (Fig. 5-23). The second technique, by far the most extensively used, employs curved surface laminography (tomography).

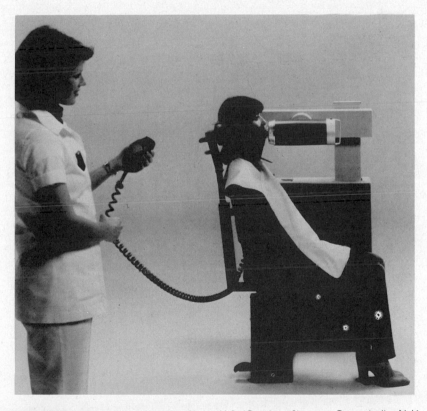

Fig. 5-23. Intraoral source Siemens Status X-2. (Courtesy Siemens Corp., Iselin, N.J.)

Tomography

Tomography (laminography) is a radiographic technique that allows radiographing structures in one plane of an object while blurring or eliminating images from structures in other planes. "Tomo" is the Greek word for section, lamina, or layer and therefore is used to describe this "layered" radiographic technique. Tomography is used extensively in medicine; the most recent advance is the "CAT scan" (computerized axial tomography).

A tomogram is made by moving the x-ray source and the film in opposite directions in a fixed relationship, through one or a series of rotation points, while the patient remains stationary (Fig. 5-24). The plane of the object that is not blurred on the radiograph is called the *plane of acceptable detail* or *focal trough*. The point or points of rotation can be inside or outside of the focal trough. The width or thickness of the focal trough is governed by many factors including the angle of movement of the x-ray beam, the width of the x-ray beam, and the size of the focal spot. Any object that lies in the focal plane will be seen clearly and objects above and below it will appear blurred. By varying the focal-object distance on a tomographic series, different focal troughs or "cuts" can be achieved. A tomographic series is usually composed of multiple cuts, 0.5 cm apart, with the number of cuts varying according to the thickness of the object.

A panoramic radiograph of the maxilla and mandible, produced by using tomography, is properly referred to as a *pantomogram*. The pantomogram is a curved surface

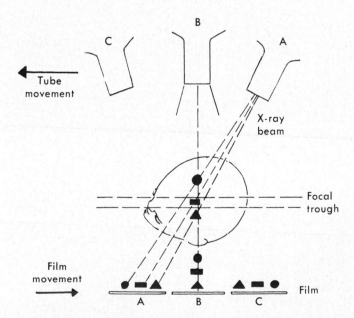

Fig. 5-24. Diagram illustrating principle of tomography. Note that only objects in focal trough *(square)* project onto the same area of the film and are not blurred out.

tomogram. In common usage the term "panoramic radiograph" is usually substituted for pantomogram.

There are many pantomographic units available. They differ primarily in the number and locations of the centers of rotation, whether there is a fixed or adjustable focal trough, and the type and shape of film transport mechanism. All units utilize intensifying screens with film size being either 5 × 12 or 6 × 12 inches. Design differences include head positioning devices, standing or sitting patient position, and wall mounting or free standing units.

Individual manufacturers use trade names such as Panorex, Orthopantomograph, Panelipse, and Panoral for their own panoramic units. Each manufacturer's machine has its own technique for operation, which can be learned easily from the unit's instruction manual (Figs. 5-25 to 5-27). With any of the pantomographic units, positioning the patient's head and maintaining that position during the movement of the tube head and the film around the patient are extremely important. If this is not done, the desired structure to be radiographed may not be in the plane of focus or the focal trough and will appear blurred on the radiograph.

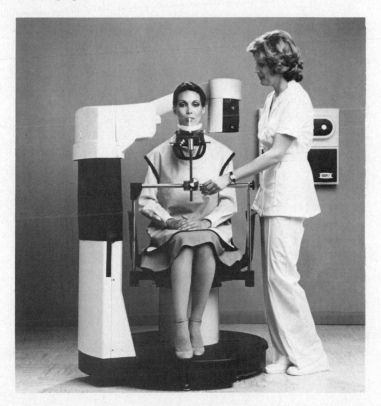

Fig. 5-25. Panorex 2 X-ray System. (Courtesy S.S. White Dental Products International, Pennwalt Corp.)

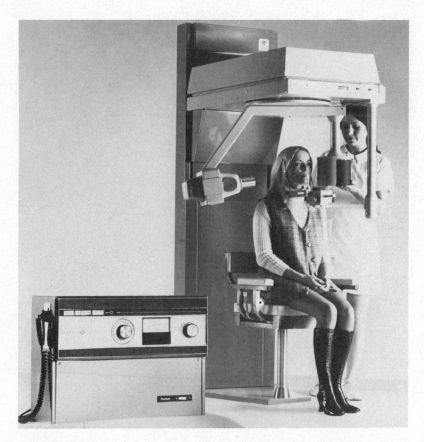

Fig. 5-26. G.E. Panelipse panoramic x-ray machine. (Courtesy General Electric Co., Milwaukee.)

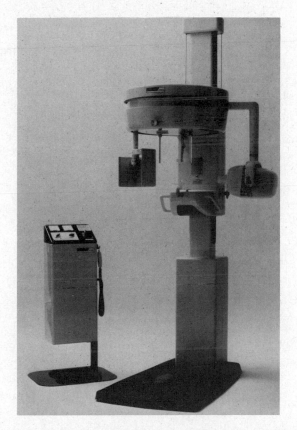

Fig. 5-27. Panoral pantomographic x-ray machine. (Courtesy Sybron Corp., Romulus, Mich.)

Advantages and disadvantages

Like any new technique, panoramic tomography has its advantages and disadvantages when compared with conventional intraoral techniques. These units are still very expensive, costing approximately four times as much as a regular x-ray tube-head, which is still necessary even with the panoramic unit. The full-mouth series, composed of periapical and bite-wing films, has been the accepted norm for routine dental radiography and any new techniques should be judged in comparison.

Advantages

Size of the area radiographed. This is one of the major advantages of the pantomograph. The full-mouth survey is not composed of radiographs of the entire mouth but the teeth, alveolar ridges, and part of the supporting structures. The pantomogram covers an area that includes all of the mandible from condyle to condyle and the maxillary regions extending superiorly to the middle third of the orbits (Fig. 5-28). Areas such as the condyles, inferior border, angle and ascending ramus of the mandible, and the entire maxillary sinus that are not visualized on intraoral surveys are seen routinely on pantomograms. Many areas of disease that might go undetected on intraoral surveys will be seen on pantomograms.

Quality control. In maintaining radiographic quality control, the full radiographic visualization of all the teeth and surrounding bone, including the third molar area, is of prime importance. The pantomograph consistently shows these areas and eliminates the need for retakes.

Simplicity. Pantomographic procedures are relatively simple to perform. With a minimum amount of training and by paying strict attention to detail, the dentist or dental auxiliary can become very proficient in taking these films.

Patient cooperation. Since pantomography is an extraoral procedure, it requires a minimum amount of patient cooperation. There is nothing placed in the patient's mouth and he is only required to stand or sit still for the 15 to 22 seconds of the exposure. Most units can be operated without radiation to demonstrate what the procedure will be like before the actual exposure is made. Pantomography virtually eliminates problems with intractable gaggers, patients with trismus, and fearful or uncooperative children.

Time. Less time is required to do a pantomographic examination than an intraoral survey. The most skilled operator requires at least 15 minutes to do an intraoral survey; pantomograms can be taken in less than 5 minutes.

Dose. There seems to be general agreement that the radiation dose to the patient is relatively low or, at most, equal to conventional intraoral radiography.[1-3] White and Weissman have reported that the dose level of pantomograph radiography might be 15% of that of a full-mouth intraoral survey.[1] A rough approximation of the patient's comparable skin doses from the two methods might be arrived at by considering the size and shape of the two x-ray beams. The conventional technique uses an x-ray beam 2¾ inches in

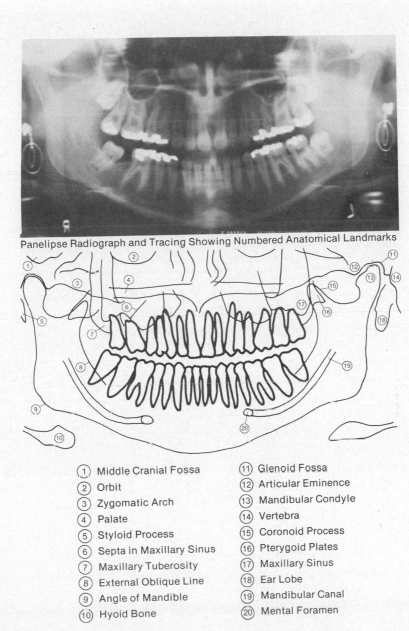

Panelipse Radiograph and Tracing Showing Numbered Anatomical Landmarks

1. Middle Cranial Fossa
2. Orbit
3. Zygomatic Arch
4. Palate
5. Styloid Process
6. Septa in Maxillary Sinus
7. Maxillary Tuberosity
8. External Oblique Line
9. Angle of Mandible
10. Hyoid Bone
11. Glenoid Fossa
12. Articular Eminence
13. Mandibular Condyle
14. Vertebra
15. Coronoid Process
16. Pterygoid Plates
17. Maxillary Sinus
18. Ear Lobe
19. Mandibular Canal
20. Mental Foramen

Fig. 5-28. Panoramic radiograph and tracing showing numbered anatomic landmarks. (Courtesy General Electric Co., Milwaukee.)

diameter and this area of exposure (circular or rectangular) is repeated across the face about 18 times for a full-mouth survey at an approximate exposure time of $^4/_{10}$ second per film. The pantomographic units use a slit-beam technique. The size of the beam, as it travels across the patient's face, is approximately 2 mm $\times$ 30 mm.

As far as the operator's exposure is concerned, at a distance of 6 feet from the patient, the exposure levels are lower than those using conventional techniques.[4]

Patient education. Pantomographic films are a valuable aid in patient education and case presentation. Patients can more easily understand conditions explained to them on pantomograms than on full-mouth surveys. Lay persons are usually confused by the multiwindowed mount of the full-mouth survey where teeth appear more than once on different projections. The panoramic view more closely resembles the pictures or illustrations that they are used to seeing. Conditions such as impactions, eruption patterns of teeth, the need for replacement of missing teeth, and fractures are more easily illustrated on panoramic views.

Disadvantages

Image quality. Tomograms inherently show magnification, geometric distortion, and poor definition.[5] Compared to intraoral radiographs the pantomogram does not give comparable radiographic definition. Besides the tomographic process, other factors that tend to degrade the images as compared to intraoral films are: (1) external placement of the film with resulting increased object-film distance, (2) the use of intensifying screens, and (3) faster film with larger grain size.

There are many diagnostic problems where a high degree of radiographic definition is essential. Such conditions as the early detection of interproximal or recurrent caries, disruptions in the lamina dura, loss of crestal alveolar bone, and a thickened periodontal membrane all require the maximum amoung of radiographic definition. These are common diagnostic problems that comprise the bulk of the diagnostic problems for practitioners and the pantomograph seems to be lacking in this requirement. If a pantomogram is to be used instead of conventional periapical films, it must be augmented with bite-wings and selective periapical films where indicated.

Focal trough (plane). Areas that lie outside of the focal trough may be seen poorly or not at all. The focal trough or plane of acceptable detail is not as wide as either the mandible or maxilla and it is only structures or changes that lie within the trough that are visualized clearly. Pantomographic units that have adjustable focal troughs have far greater diagnostic capabilities than those that do not.

Overlap. Pantomographic units have a tendency to produce overlapping of the teeth images most particularly in the premolar area.

Superimposition. There is very often superimposition of the spinal column on the anterior portion of the pantomogram. Theoretically, if the patient is positioned perfectly this will not happen. However, all patients are not perfect and some have physical problems that make positioning difficult. The anterior teeth and periapical bone are the most difficult areas to interpret on pantomograms.

Distortion. The amount of vertical and horizontal distortion varies from one part of the film to another. This results in an uneven magnification of the image; structures and spaces may seem larger than they actually are.

Overuse. This is one of the prime concerns in regard to patient dosage. The ease and convenience in obtaining the pantomograph might lead to carelessness by substitution for other projections that might be adequate. The pantomogram might be taken because it is easier to do than taking one periapical film of an area.

Processing

Panoramic films are processed in regular dental solutions. Time-temperature technique is essential, because the film is extremely sensitive. As previously mentioned, proper safelighting should be maintained.

STUDY QUESTIONS

1. Explain why it is necessary to use occlusal films in localizing impacted teeth.
2. List three indications for using extraoral views in dentistry.
3. Which extraoral projection is most diagnostic for maxillary sinus pathologic conditions. How is this film taken?
4. What extra precautions must be taken in the darkroom when loading cassettes and processing extraoral films?
5. Why is correct positioning of the patient's head so important in pantomographic radiology?
6. How can one differentiate the left side of the patient from the right on an extraoral radiograph?
7. If a periapical film of an impacted mandibular third molar cannot be positioned so the complete root can be seen, what would you do?
8. What projection would you use to localize a foreign body in the floor of the mouth?
9. What areas of the maxilla and mandible are not shown on the pantomographic radiograph?
10. Is pantomographic or bite-wing film more diagnostic for caries? Why?

REFERENCES

1. White, S.C., and Weissman, D.: Relative discernment of lesions by intraoral and panoramic radiography, J. Am. Dent. Assoc., December **95**:117, 1977.
2. Van Aken, J., and Vander Linden, L.W.: The integral absorbed dose in conventional and panoramic complete examination, Oral Surg. **22**:603, November 1966.
3. Valachovic, R.W., and Lurie, A.G.: Risk benefit considerations in pedodontic radiology, Pediatr. Dent. **2**:128, 1980.
4. Brueggeman, I.A.: Evaluation of a Panorex unit, Oral Surg. **24**:348, September 1967.
5. Reports of councils and bureaus, J. Am. Dent. Assoc. **94**:147, January 1977.

chapter 6 Patient management and special problems

MANAGEMENT

The area of patient management is as important to the dental auxiliary as it is to the dentist. Included in patient management are assignments such as scheduling appointments, handling and screening telephone calls, collecting fees, and most importantly using patient psychology.

The dental auxiliary will encounter all types of personalities in the dental office. Some patients may be very apprehensive and tense about dental treatment while others may be calm and very matter-of-fact in attitude. Some patients will reveal their anxieties in behavioral and speech patterns; others may hide them. Even with modern equipment, techniques, and attitudes, dentistry still remains a stressful procedure for the majority of patients.

One of the important roles of the dental auxiliary, which performed successfully will make the work easier, is to try to relax the patient and make him feel at ease. The dental auxiliary may be the first member of the office staff to greet the patient in the reception area. Patients like to be recognized and greeted by name. This is especially important for new patients. It is helpful to say "We will be with you shortly" rather than "The doctor will be with you shortly." "We" implies the team concept of treatment and stresses the importance of the dental auxiliary in the office.

In performing dental radiography the dental auxiliary also must develop a chairside manner. Patients must be made to feel comfortable and confident in the auxiliary's ability to perform the radiographic examination.

With the expanding role of the dental auxiliary, more and more dental offices are utilizing auxiliaries to do radiographic surveys. However, there are many patients who have never had dental auxiliaries perform any services for them. They are accustomed to having the dentist do all their work. These patients may be apprehensive and even object to the auxiliary's performing any service for them. This attitude should not be taken personally; it should be regarded as a lack of patient orientation to new modes of treatment. If the patient objects strenuously, the dentist should be called in to reassure him. The dental auxiliary should then perform the procedure.

We are striving for high clinical proficiency, with efficient and confident work patterns. These objectives can be achieved through experience and critical evaluation by oneself, co-workers, and the dentist.

When seating the patient and draping him with the lead apron, some small talk may help to relax him. Patients want to know that you are interested in them and not just performing a mechanical procedure. This is not wasted time, as a relaxed, confident patient is much easier to work with.

Appearance is very important. The dental auxiliary should wear a clean uniform daily and be well groomed. Some dentists insist that their auxiliaries wear caps, and they object to long, flowing hair in the treatment room. Remember to wash your hands after the patient is seated in the dental chair so that the patient can take note of this hygienic procedure. If you sneeze, cough, pick up something from the floor, or have to leave the treatment room, hands should be rewashed before starting work again.

Never chew gum while working with patients; if you must smoke, it should be remembered that tobacco odor on breath or hands can be very offensive to patients. Mouthwash and hand lotions can be used to mask the tobacco residue before seeing patients.

Always explain to the patient what procedures you are going to perform and indicate how many films will be taken. Answer any questions the patient has if you feel capable of doing so. If the question involves diagnostic judgments or treatment planning it should be referred to the doctor. Patients will often ask about the need for radiographs and the potential radiation hazards. Since these questions are usually asked before work begins, a well-answered question will give the patient confidence and lessen his apprehension about having the radiographs taken by a dental auxiliary. It is hoped that answers to questions of this type will be found in this text.

The "light touch" of certain dentists and dental auxiliaries is really nothing more than good technique developed with experience and respect for the oral tissues. No one is born with a "heavy hand," and thus there is no excuse for clumsy, uncomfortable intraoral radiographic technique.

Films must be placed in the patient's mouth and directions given to the patient in a manner that indicates self-confidence. A patient likes to feel that the operator is in full control of the situation at all times. If a finger-holding technique is used, when guiding the patient's finger to support the film, grasp his hand firmly and guide it into place decisively. Instructions to the patient should be given in a firm but polite tone. Words of encouragement and praise for the patient's cooperation should be used. If a patient is not following instructions, for example, raising his head and altering occlusal plane orientation, the patient should be corrected. Do not accept improper patient position because you are too reticent to remind him about his movements.

Every patient is different, both in the anatomic configuration of his mouth and in his psychologic makeup. This is the challenge of the profession: to be able to perform one's duties and to maintain standards of excellence although the clinical situation may change. Through study, practice, and self-evaluation, these goals can be met.

SPECIAL PROBLEMS

Gagging

Of all the problems one may encounter in intraoral radiography, gagging is probably the most troublesome. Gagging, or more properly the gag reflex, is a body defense mechanism. The coughing and retching produced in the gag reflex are meant to expel any foreign body from the throat and thus protect the airway from obstruction. The anesthesiologist never leaves his patient after surgery with a general anesthetic until the patient is awake and his gag reflex restored. At this point the patient can expel any mucus or other material that might obstruct the air passage because of the action of the gag reflex.

All patients have gag reflexes. The level of excitation of these reflexes varies from person to person. It is the patient with the low threshold for stimulation of the gag reflex who presents the problem in intraoral radiography.

There are very few patients, probably less than 0.1%, whose gag reflex is so active that intraoral radiography is impossible. With this in mind, how do we deal with the remaining 99.9%? The following are a set of generally accepted suggestions and techniques that should be used to prevent gagging and to overcome it when it occurs. Not all techniques are applicable, nor will they succeed with every patient. One must be able to determine which technique will best suit the individual patient.

Attitude. Always give the appearance of being in control of the situation. The patient wants to believe that the operator is so competent that it would be impossible for the film to slip and lodge in his throat. Firm positioning of the film and the patient's holding finger, with decisive vocal instructions to the patient, is necessary.

Think positively; never mention the possibility of gagging. The worst thing you can say to a patient is, "This won't make you gag." The patient may never have thought of gagging until reminded of the possibility.

Film order and technique. When taking a full-mouth radiographic survey, start in the maxilla, taking the anterior films first and working posteriorly. The film placement in the maxillary molar area is the one most likely to excite the gag reflex. Once the reflex is excited, the patient may continue to gag even on anterior films.

When placing the film in the patient's mouth for maxillary molars and premolars, do not slide the film along the palate. Place the film in the desired position on the lingual surface of the teeth, and then with one decisive motion bring the film into contact with the palate.

Always set the timing dial for the desired exposure before you place the film in the patient's mouth. Have the tube on the side of the patient's face that is to be radiographed, with the PID at the approximate vertical angulation. The object is to minimize the amount of time the film packet has to remain in the patient's mouth. Preparations like these can save valuable seconds and lessen the likelihood of the patient's gagging. Generally, the longer the film stays in the mouth, the more likelihood of gagging.

Deep breathing. It is often helpful to instruct the patient to take deep breaths through his nose while the film packet is being placed in a gag-sensitive area such as the palate. Why this works is debatable, but it may be that breathing through the nose avoids the rush of air across the sensitive tissues of the palate. Another explanation is that it gives the patient something to do and may distract him from thinking about gagging. Use a firm tone of voice when instructing the patient to take these deep breaths. The operator may also take some audible deep breaths to encourage the patient to do likewise.

Bite blocks and film-holding devices. Any film-holding device that requires the patient to bite and maintain pressure may also be helpful in avoiding gagging. Again, the patient is given something positive to do. Another tactile sensation, that of biting and the pressure of the bite block against the teeth, may distract the patient from thoughts of gagging.

Lozenges, gargles, and sprays. All of these may be of some help in certain situations. It is most important that the patient be made to believe that the medication will have an effect. There have been instances where a vitamin pill was given to a patient as an antigag pill. The patient was told in advance what the pill would do, and the rate of success was very high. This placebo effect is seen also in many other areas of dental practice. Note, however, that the patient was told what the effect of the placebo medication would be.

There are many viscous topical anesthetics available for rinsing the mouth, gargling, or spraying the palate to produce a numbing sensation and hopefully block the gag reflex.

An undiluted mouthwash may also have some anesthetic effects on the palate. Many cough lozenges contain some local anesthetic; having the patient suck on a lozenge before radiography may be helpful.

In all these cases it may not be so much the anesthetic vehicle used as the manner of presentation to the patient that produces the desired results.

Hypnosis. Although the practice of hypnosis is out of the province of the dental auxiliary its use in dentistry should be mentioned. In intractable gaggers hypnosis by trained, competent practitioners may be necessary to permit intraoral radiography.

It should be pointed out that convincing a patient that something (like gagging) may not occur can be considered a form of hypnosis. An application of this principle is to tell the gagging patient that you are going to press the antigag nerve located in his neck. We know that there is no antigag nerve, but the patient may not. If the area in the neck is pressed hard, some sensation will occur and the patient may become convinced that gagging will not occur.

Salt. One of the more amusing techniques described in the literature to stop gagging is to place ordinary table salt on the tip of the tongue of the gagging patient. The salt is placed in the palm of the patient's hand and he is asked to touch the tip of his tongue to the salt and then raise the tongue to touch the palate. It may be a method worth trying at least once in one's professional career.

For the intractable gagger, when all else fails, one must then resort to auxiliary technique. The panoramic film, previously discussed, has the advantage of circumventing the gag reflex.

171

Localization

Standard intraoral periapical and bite-wing films show the teeth and bone in only two dimensions—the superoinferior and anteroposterior plane. There are, however, many clinical situations when it is necessary for a proper radiographic diagnosis to establish the position of structures in the buccolingual plane. An example of this type would be the localization of the impacted canine seen in Fig. 6-1. The location of the impaction is essential information that is needed by the surgeon in planning the incision.

The four techniques that can be used for localization are: (1) definition evaluation, (2) tube shift, (3) right-angle technique, and (4) pantomography.

Definition evaluation. Structures that lie closer to the x-ray film will have better radiographic definition than those that are farther from the film. This is true for both intraoral and extraoral films. It is sometimes possible, depending on the quality of the radiograph, to determine the relative position of superimposed structures by determining which has better radiographic definition. Because intraoral film is positioned lingually in the patient's mouth, the superimposed structure that is more sharply defined will be positioned lingually in relation to the other structures (Fig. 6-2). An advantage of this technique, when compared to the others that follow, is that it requires no further x-ray exposures of the patient.

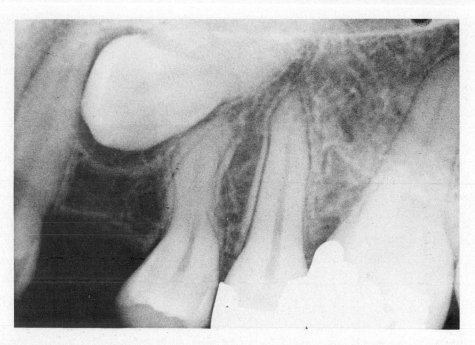

Fig. 6-1. Impacted maxillary canine. Is the tooth positioned bucally or palatally to the alveolar ridge?

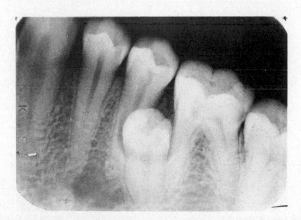

Fig. 6-2. Localization of definition. Is the impacted supernumerary tooth more clearly defined than the rest of the teeth? If not, it is probably positioned buccally.

173

Tube shift. The tube shift method uses what has been referred to as ''Clark's rule'' or the ''buccal object rule.'' Its advantage is that localization can be accomplished by using standard periapical technique. To define the buccolingual relationship between two structures that appear radiologically superimposed, a second radiograph is taken. All factors remain the same for the second exposure except the tube is shifted about 20 degrees in either the vertical or the horizontal angulation. When the two radiographs are compared, the buccal object will appear to have moved in the opposite direction from the tube shift (Figs. 6-3 and 6-4). If the tube is shifted mesially by changing the horizontal angulation, the buccal object will appear to have moved distally. In the mandible, for example, if the vertical angulation is increased by moving the beam down, the buccal object will appear to have moved superiorly on the film. The key phrase is ''buccal opposite'' when using the buccal object rule.

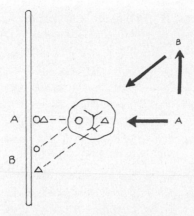

Fig. 6-3. Buccal object rule. As the tube position is shifted mesially (position *B*), the buccal object is seen to move relatively in the opposite direction, distally.

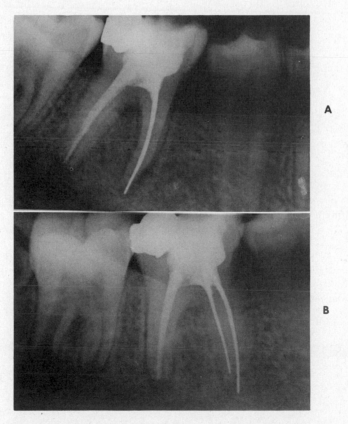

A

B

Fig. 6-4. Radiographs illustrating the buccal-object rule. The tube in *B* was shifted to the mesial indicating that the short endodontic point is in the mesiobuccal canal.

175

Right-angle technique. The right-angle technique, utilizing occlusal film, is discussed in detail in Chapter 5.

Pantomography. The redundant images produced in the anterior region by some pantomographic units, such as the Panorex unit, can be used to localize objects in that area. In viewing the film, the object in question will be seen twice, once on each half of the film. A recommended technique is to compare the relative movement of the object to adjacent structures from one side of the film to the other with the direction that the clinician reads the film (for example, left to right).[1] The object will seem to have moved in the same direction as the clinicans viewing movement if it is lingually positioned, and the opposite direction if it is on the buccal side (Fig. 6-5).

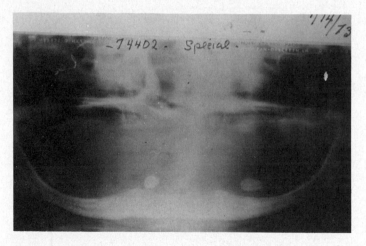

Fig. 6-5. Localization of an object by pantomographic redundant image.

Third molars

The third molars are in an area of the mouth difficult to radiograph. In many cases it may not be possible to position the film packet intraorally to visualize these areas adequately on radiographs. This is especially true if the teeth are impacted. In these cases it may be necessary to utilize the extraoral and panoramic techniques described in Chapter 5.

Maxilla. As the film is placed more and more distally to the patient's throat, the likelihood of exciting the gag reflex increases. It may be helpful to hold the film packet in a hemostat so as to maintain a minimum of contact with the palate. The film packet should be kept as parallel to the palatal vault as possible. To avoid distortion the vertical angulation will have to be increased, with the resulting relationship of the central ray to the film packet looking very much like an occlusal projection.

Mandible. The most common difficulty in radiographing lower third molars is the inability to place the film packet distal enough to record the image of the whole tooth and root structure. This placement is prevented by the muscles of the floor of the mouth and tongue.

To overcome this problem the tongue can be deflected to the opposite side of the mouth by the operator's finger or a mouth mirror. The floor of the mouth is gently depressed, almost massaged, to relax the mylohyoid muscle. While this is being done the film packet is slid along the lingual surface of the mandible as far distally as possible. In certain horizontal impactions of the mandible it may be necessary to distort the image in the horizontal plane in order to visualize the entire tooth with intraoral radiography. This is done by changing the horizontal angulation of the x-ray beam so that it is not at right angles to the film packet, which is the usual procedure, but so that the beam comes from the distal side and the central ray makes an acute angle with the film.

Narrow arch

In some mouths it may be impossible to place anterior film packets properly without excessive bending, with resultant distortion of the radiographic image. The best way to overcome this problem is to vary the film size. There is no rule that you cannot use different sized intraoral packets in the same full-mouth series. The only possible problem will be in mounting the films. The smaller or narrower films will have to be attached to the mount by cellophane tape or staples so they do not slip from the window in the mount. Pedodontic or narrow film may be used as the situation dictates (Fig. 6-6).

If radiographs show overlapping of teeth, especially in the anterior region, it does not necessarily indicate that the films were taken improperly. If the teeth are overlapped in the mouth, they will appear overlapped radiographically.

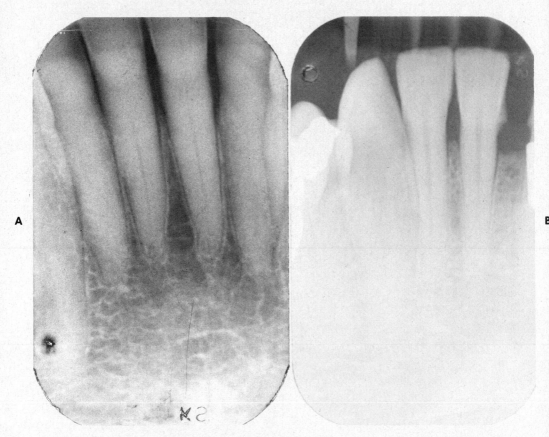

A   B

Fig. 6-6. Periapical radiographs of lower anterior region using **A,** child size (#0), and **B,** narrow anterior (#1) film.

Shallow palate

The shallow palatal vault presents the greatest problem in the paralleling technique. Because of the bony structures it may be impossible to place the film packet parallel to the long axis of the tooth and yet be high enough to record the radiographic image (Fig. 6-7). This technique may have to be abandoned for these patients and the bisecting-angle technique used instead.

In the bisecting-angle technique the shallow palate is compensated for by increasing the vertical angulation. As long as the film packet is in the patient's mouth so that there is a 3 mm border projecting beneath the incisal or occlusal edge of the teeth and the central ray bisects the angle formed between film packet and the long axis of the tooth, the shallow palate will be compensated for (Fig. 6-8).

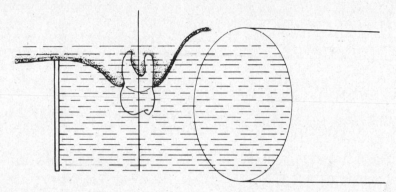

Fig. 6-7. Problem of film placement in paralleling technique with patients with low palatal vaults. Note that film cannot be placed high enough to record image of root apices.

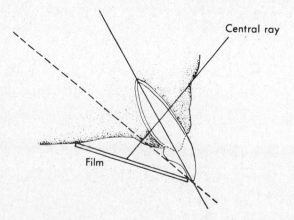

Fig. 6-8. How to overcome the problem of a low palatal vault in bisecting-angle technique. Note increase in vertical angulation.

179

Lingual frenulum

It is extremely difficult to radiograph patients who have a large, tight, lingual frenulum, attached close to the tip of the tongue. These patients are sometimes referred to as "tongue tied" because they cannot protrude their tongues very far out of their mouths.

The paralleling technique is not the method of choice for these patients because the tight frenulum will not allow placement of the film packet deep in the floor of the mouth. Relaxing the muscle as recommended for the mylohyoid will still not produce enough room. It is best to use the bisecting technique. Since the film cannot be placed very deep in the mouth, negative vertical angulations in the range of $-40°$ to $-60°$ can be expected.

Tori

The maxillary torus (torus palatinus) if present usually presents no problems in periapical radiography. It is located posteriorly in the midline of the palate and does not hinder film placement. The best way to radiograph a torus palatinus is by use of an occlusal projection.

The mandibular tori, or torus as the case may be, are located on the lingual aspect of the mandible in the premolar area. Their presence prevents the placement of the film packet in its usual position. This difficulty is more accentuated in the bisecting-angle technique than in the paralleling technique. The film packet cannot be depressed into the floor of the mouth while being kept close to the lingual surface of the teeth. The only possible solution is to place the film over the torus. This increases the angle between the film packet and the long axis of the tooth and is compensated for by increasing the vertical angulation to bisect the angle.

Canine overlap

Overlapping the image of the mesial portion of the maxillary first premolar with the image of the distal surface of the canine is a common problem. The overlapping is caused by the large palatal cusp of the first premolar. The problem can be solved by changing the horizontal angulation so that the central ray comes more from the distal side, as in a premolar periapical projection (Fig. 6-9); then the palatal cusp will not be superimposed. Overlapping does not occur in the mandible because the first premolar has a very small lingual cusp.

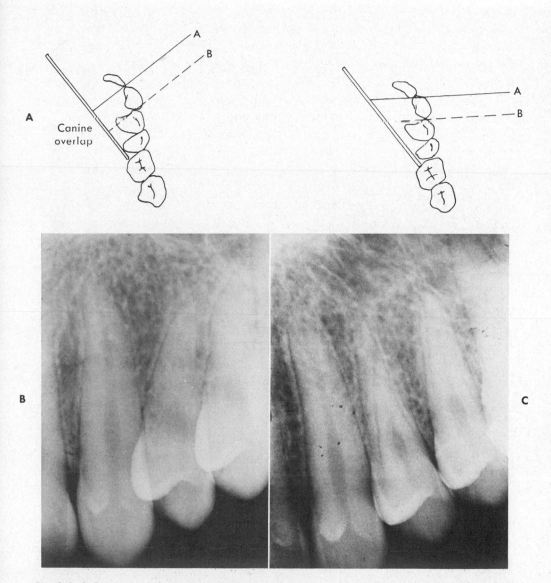

Fig. 6-9. A, Diagram of changing horizontal angulation to avoid distal overlap of maxillary canine. **B,** Overlapped canine. **C,** Overlapping eliminated.

Grid measurement

Intraoral measurement grids are available that superimpose radiopaque thin lines in the vertical and horizontal planes in 1-mm gradations. The measurement grid is affixed to the front of the film packet when the exposure is made. No increase in exposure is necessary with the use of this marking grid. The measurement grid should not be confused with the grid used in extraoral projections (Chapter 5) to absorb object scatter (Figs. 6-10 and 6-11).

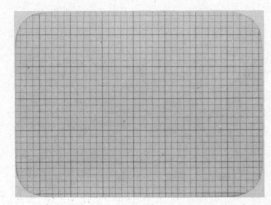

Fig. 6-10. Photograph of intraoral grid that is placed on dental film packet.

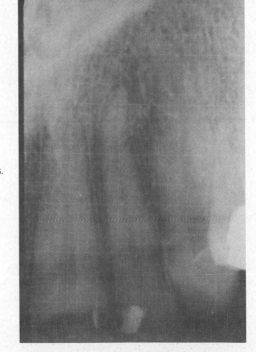

Fig. 6-11. Radiograph with grid markings.

Radiopaque media

The use of radiopaque media has many applications in dental practice. It is used routinely in endodontics, with the radiopaque file, to determine root length. Gutta-percha or silver points can be placed in periodontal soft tissue pockets to determine pocket depth and direction. Fistulous tracts can be traced to their origin using thin, flexible wire or gutta-percha points (Fig. 6-12).

The technique of sialography involves injecting radiopaque media into salivary ducts and glands and then visualizing these soft tissues radiographically. This method is used in diagnosing ductal and glandular obstructions, salivary stones, infections, and tumors of the major salivary glands. The contrast medium used is usually an iodine containing formula in either an aqueous or oil suspension (Fig. 6-13).

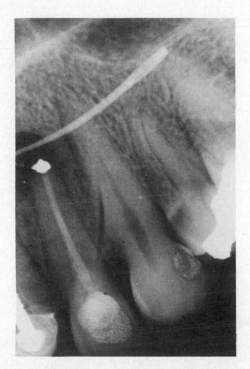 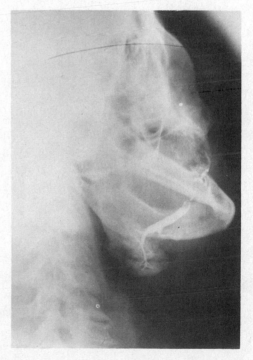

Fig. 6-12. Fistulous tract traced back from palatal opening to its origin by inertion of gutta-percha point.

Fig. 6-13. Sialograph outlining submandibular duct and gland.

183

Trismus

Trismus is the condition with which a patient is unable to open his mouth. It may be partial or complete and is usually caused by infection or trauma. To make an adequate diagnosis and identify the infected tooth or area, radiographs are necessary. If the patient's mouth cannot be opened at all, extraoral or panoramic films will be necessary. If there is partial opening, it may be possible to place an intraoral film by modifying the usual technique. A hemostat is used to hold the film packet since it is much narrower than a finger or any other film-holding device. The film packet is placed in the mouth by sliding it between the partially opened anterior teeth in the horizontal plane. Once beyond the teeth, the film can be turned to its proper vertical orientation. The patient then holds the hemostat with the film packet attached to it in position while the exposure is made.

Positive medical history

Rubber gloves should always be worn while radiographing patients with a positive medical history of syphilis or other contagious diseases transmitted by contact. The old adage about an ounce of prevention could never be more applicable. If the operator is at all suspicious because of the patient's history or lesions present in the patient's mouth, gloves should be worn. These gloves are made in disposable form and are easily obtained from dental suppliers.

Handicapped patients

The problems in treating the handicapped patient in the dental office vary according to the degree of disability. With patients confined to wheelchairs it may be easier to radiograph them in the wheelchair than to transfer them to the dental chair. This presents no problem as long as the x-ray machine and patient can be maneuvered into the proper relationship.

The patient who has no digital control cannot hold film packets in place, so a bite block or other film-holding device is used.

It is the spastic patient with uncontrollable movements who presents the greatest problem. It may be necessary for someone, usually a parent or friend, to hold the patient's head steady while the radiograph is being taken. This person can wear lead gloves and a lead apron for radiation protection. It should not be the dental auxiliary, who constantly works with radiation, holding the patient and standing in the direct x-ray beam.

In the totally unmanageable patient, radiographs may have to be taken with the patient under general anesthesia. These films are usually developed immediately and the necessary dental procedures performed while the patient is still anesthetized.

Bedridden patients

There may be patients in hospitals and nursing homes who cannot be brought to the dental suites and for whom dental procedures and radiographs must be done at the bedside. Mobile dental x-ray units can be brought to the bed and radiographs taken. For the patient in the supine position, it is easier to use a film-holding device with a localizing ring. In treating a patient at home or at a site that does not have a dental x-ray unit, there are portable x-ray units that can be adapted for dental use and assembled on site (Fig. 6-14). A small, portable, rapid processing tank should also be brought along so that the radiographs can be processed and the patient treated at the same visit.

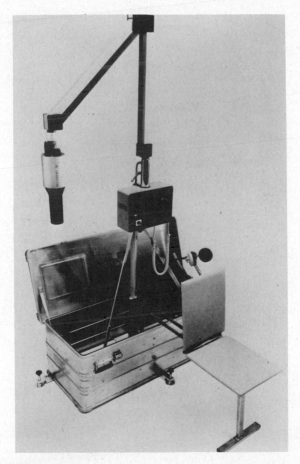

Fig. 6-14. Siemens Portaray transportable x-ray examination unit. (Courtesy Siemens Corp., Iselin, N.J.)

Children

In dental radiography the complete cooperation of the patient is necessary. If the patient moves, the radiographic image will be blurred and the film rendered useless. In no other area of dentistry is this absolute cooperation necessary. If a child moves during an operative dentistry procedure it can be compensated for. In radiography the patient must hold still while the exposure is being made.

To any child the unknown is a frightening thing, and very few children know anything about x-rays. In fact, the dental radiograph may be their first introduction to any radiography. The procedure then must be explained to the child in terms he can understand. One should talk of taking a ''picture'' of the tooth with a ''camera.'' Remind the child that he must hold still when the picture is being taken. Show the child the film packet and let him put in in his mouth. Taking a picture of the child's thumb is a good way to introduce the concept of holding still and to assure the child that he will feel nothing when the tooth is radiographed. Of course, the x-ray machine is off when these thumb exposures are made.

Children like to see pictures, and it is sometimes helpful to show the child what a radiograph of a tooth looks like. This is followed by the promise of showing the child what his teeth will look like on the finished radiograph. We have, in certain instances, even taken the child into the darkroom and let him help process the films. Children are fascinated by the darkroom with its tanks and chemicals. Any effort expended to relax the child and make him feel at ease will reap benefits at later appointments.

Children usually tolerate periapical films very well and can hold them in place with the thumb or bite block. If these is resistance to holding the film, have the child bite on the film and then increase the vertical angulation to bisect the angle so it appears that you are almost taking an occlusal projection (Fig. 6-15). This type of film is not as desirable as the regular technique, but it is better than no film at all. This method will work for any area of the child's mouth, and a full-mouth series can be taken this way if necessary. Either adult size or occlusal film can be used for this technique (Fig. 6-16).

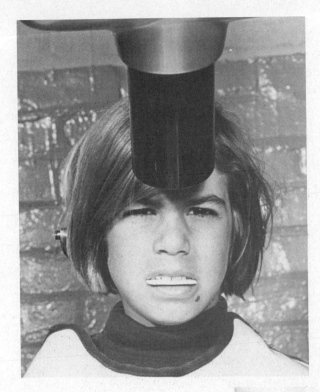

Fig. 6-15. Technique for periapical films that allows child to bite on film. Note increase in vertical angulation.

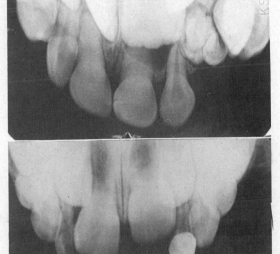

A

B

Fig. 6-16. Radiographs taken by having the child bite the film packet. **A,** Adult size periapical film packet. (Note odontoma blocking tooth eruption.) **B,** Occlusal film packet.

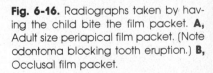

Reverse bite-wings. Some children will not tolerate the placement of the bite-wing film. When instructed to close on the tab they push the lower part of the film out of the floor of the mouth with the tongue and then close their teeth on the film. If after repeated attempts proper placement meets with failure, a reverse bite-wing technique can be substituted. In this method the film packet is placed on the cheek side of the teeth in the buccal sulcus (Fig. 6-17). The child bites on the tab to hold the film packet in place. The x-ray beam is directed extraorally from under the opposite side of the mandible as in a lateral oblique projection (Fig. 6-18). The exposure time must be increased by a factor of 4 or 5 because of the increased FFD. The resulting film will not have the detail of an intraoral bite-wing radiograph but will be a useful substitute (Fig. 6-19).

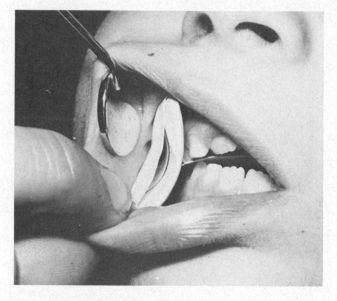

Fig. 6-17. Film placement for reverse bite-wing radiograph.

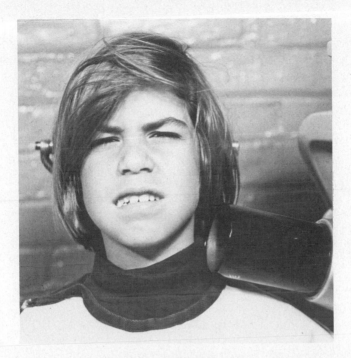

Fig. 6-18. Tube position for reverse bite-wing radiograph. Note that central ray is directed from underneath mandible of opposite side while being aimed at bite-wing film.

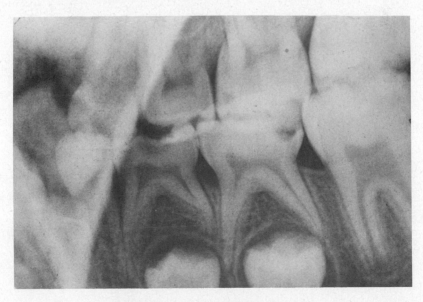

Fig. 6-19. Reverse bite-wing radiograph.

If intraoral film placement is not possible for the child, an extraoral film can be substituted. The view that is most diagnostic is a slight variation of the lateral oblique technique. The cassette is positioned in the same way, but the central ray is directed from behind the angle of the mandible on the opposite side (Fig. 6-20). Again the radiograph is not as diagnostic as an intraoral film but better than none (Fig. 6-21).

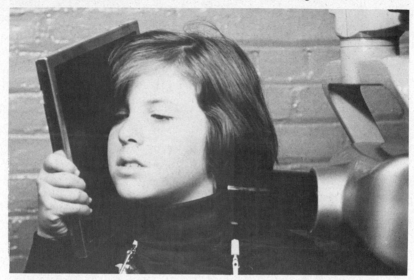

Fig. 6-20. Lateral oblique technique for caries and pathology detection in children. Note that central ray is aimed from behind angle of mandible on opposite side.

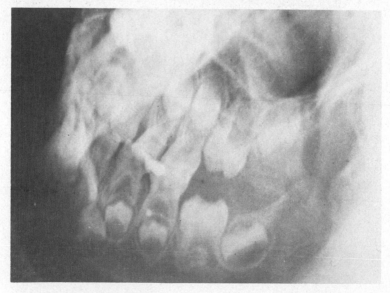

Fig. 6-21. Radiograph taken by lateral oblique technique.

If there is no extraoral cassette in the office, a piece of occlusal film can be substituted (Fig. 6-22). An exposure time of nearly 2 seconds will be necessary because of the increased FFD. The radiograph produced will be of some diagnostic value (Fig. 6-23).

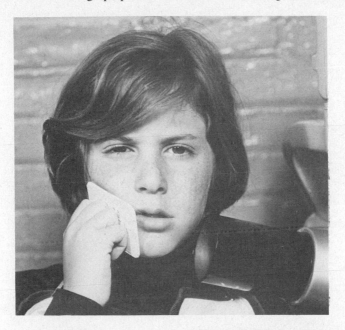

Fig. 6-22. Occlusal film packet used as extraoral film.

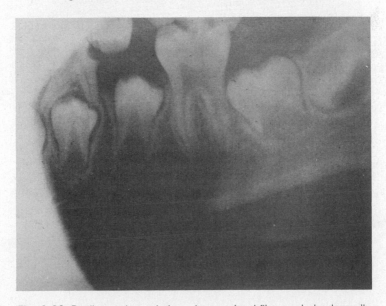

Fig. 6-23. Radiograph made by using occlusal film packet extraorally.

Taking radiographs with a rubber dam in place

In patients undergoing endodontic treatment, it is necessary to take working and measurement films while the rubber dam is in place. The bisecting method can be used with the patient supporting the film packet under the rubber dam with a finger. It is difficult to use the paralleling method with the dam in place because of the lack of working space in the mouth and the patient's inability to bite on any film-holding device because of the rubber dam clamp and protruding endodontic files from the tooth. It is best to disengage the rubber dam frame, keeping the saliva ejector in place, and position the film packet in a hemostat or Rinn ''Snap-a-Ray,'' parallel to the tooth and held by the patient.

Plastic rubber dam frames and saliva ejectors should be used to avoid superimposition of their images on the radiograph (Fig. 6-24). It is helpful to punch a hole in a predetermined corner of the dam so it will be easy to reorient the dam in the frame once the exposure had been made.

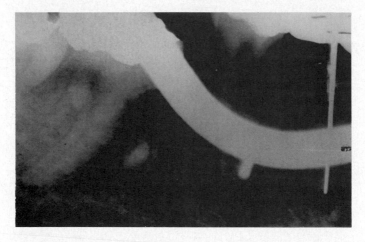

Fig. 6-24. Radiograph with superimposition of rubber dam frame.

STUDY QUESTIONS

1. What is the role of the dental auxiliary in patient management?
2. Describe the personal hygienic procedure in dental radiography of which the dental auxiliary should be aware.
3. How can the dental auxiliary convey a feeling of confidence to the patient?
4. What do you do in a situation where a patient refuses to be radiographed?
5. Why is it important for the dental auxiliary to be able to discuss radiation hazards with the patient?
6. Outline some methods that may be employed to prevent patient gagging.
7. What is the usual problem in intraoral radiography of impacted maxillary and mandibular third molars?
8. When and why should rubber gloves be worn for intraoral radiography?
9. Why is the shallow palate more of a problem in the paralleling technique than in the bisecting-angle technique?
10. What is the reverse bite-wing technique?
11. List some methods that might be used to orient a new child patient to the use of dental x-ray.
12. What is the proper film order when taking a full-mouth radiographic survey? Why?
13. What are some of the reasons that may make it impossible to take intraoral films?
14. If intraoral films cannot be taken, what should be done? Why?
15. How do exposure times of extraoral films compare with intraoral film exposure times?

REFERENCE

1. Langlais, R.P., Langland, O.E., and Morris, C.R.: Radiographic localization techniques, Dent. Radiogr. Photogr. 52:4, 1979.

chapter 7 The darkroom

The darkroom is one of the areas in a dental office for which the dental auxiliary has complete responsibility. In addition to processing film the auxiliary must keep the darkroom clean, change solutions regularly, and keep accurate records of radiographs processed. Only through meticulous attention to detail can proper darkroom technique be maintained. It is important to realize that the processing of films is a vital link in the production of the diagnostic radiograph. Errors in the darkroom can easily ruin what would otherwise have been good films, making it necessary to retake the films with the resultant loss of time and increased radiation exposure to the patient. Good chairside radiographic technique must be coupled with good darkroom technique.

The lack of attention with and concern for film processing in some dental offices is documented by reports in the literature. A study of radiographs submitted to an insurance company for reimbursement reported that a majority of the radiographs were substandard.[1] Of the radiographs judged unsatisfactory, 20% were found so because of poor density or improper processing. Another study done on film processing procedures in private offices reported some disturbing findings.[2] Severe light leaks were found in 10% of the darkrooms and about 15% of the offices changed their processing solutions less frequently than recommended. Over 40% of the darkrooms did not have a thermostat and 20% did not have a timer. As might be expected, it was shown that offices using the sight development technique had a higher mR exposure per film than offices using the time-temperature technique.

DESIGN AND REQUIREMENTS OF THE DARKROOM

The darkroom is that room in the dental office set aside from the processing of radiographs. It should be an area used only for that purpose and should not be combined with a dental laboratory or used as a lounge. The essential requirements and components of a darkroom are that it should be light-tight and have safelight and white light illumination, processing tanks, a thermostatically controlled supply of water, thermometer, timer, film racks, drying racks, and storage space.

Location and size

A properly planned and located darkroom is an important but often overlooked feature in a dental office. Darkrooms are placed in unutilized spaces, closets, and laboratories without proper concern for the function or importance of the procedures to be done in them.

It is important for the dental auxiliary to have some knowledge of planning, although in most instances they will be working in previously established facilities. However, office renovations and practice relocations occur frequently and the knowledgeable auxiliary can have valuable input in the planning and design of a new office.

The darkroom should be a space unto itself and located near the rooms where the x-ray units are placed. This will eliminate the necessity of personnel walking the entire length of the office with wet readings, thereby saving time, eliminating dripping of processing solutions, and reducing office traffic.

The darkroom should be a minimum of 16 square feet (4 × 4), allowing enough room for one person to work comfortably. The factors that should be considered in determining the space needed are: (1) the volume of radiographs to be processed, (2) the number of auxiliaries who will be doing the processing, (3) the type of processing to be done (manual, automatic, or both), and (4) space for duplicating, drying, and storage.

The walls of the darkroom should be a light color that will reflect the safelighting; darkroom walls do not have to be painted black. The surface of the walls and floor should be of a material that will resist and be cleaned of the processing solutions that will inevitably be spilled or splashed on them.

The darkroom must be completely light-tight so that when the safelight is on it is the only illumination in the darkroom. Since x-ray film is sensitive to white light, any light leaks will fog the film. A fogged film is less diagnostic and in some cases may be completely useless. The easiest way to check for light leaks is to stand in the darkroom in complete darkness; any leaks around doors will be apparent. The darkroom door should have an inside lock so that the door cannot be opened inadvertently while films are being loaded.

Lighting

There should be five different light sources in a well-designed darkroom: (1) an illuminating safelight, (2) an overhead white light, (3) a viewing safelight, (4) an x-ray viewbox, and (5) an outside warning light.

Illuminating safelight. When film packets are being opened, attached to racks, or processed safelight conditions must be maintained. As previously mentioned, white light will fog x-ray film. *Safelight* is any illumination that will not affect the x-ray film (Fig. 7-1). Not all red lights can be considered safe. The determining factors are the sensitivity to light of the x-ray film being used, as well as the position and intensity of the light source being used. Usually a 10- or 15-watt bulb with a red filter, placed 3 to 4 feet from the working surface, is used. A simple and reliable test of a safelight is to place a coin on an unwrapped, unexposed piece of dental film under safelight conditions. After 3 minutes of exposure to the safelight, the film is developed. If there is an outline of the coin on the film, the red light is not safe; the uncovered part of the film should have been as unaffected as the part covered by the coin (Fig. 7-2).

With the recent advent of newer, less light-sensitive periapical film, it has been possible to increase the safelight illumination in the darkroom. However, panoramic and other extraoral films do not have this decreased sensitivity to light and require less illumination in the darkroom. Therefore in an office where both intraoral and extraoral films are used it may be necessary to have two safelights of different intensity.

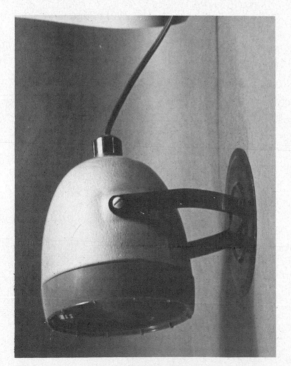

Fig. 7-1. Safelight mounted on wall of darkroom. This light is placed 3 to 4 feet from working surface and has a 10-watt bulb with a 6B Wratten filter.

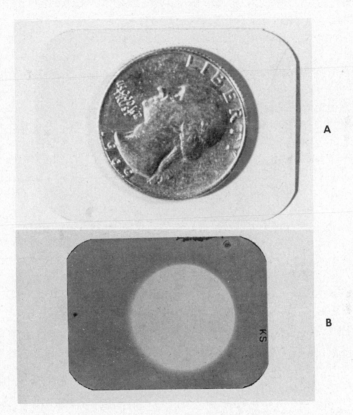

A

B

Fig. 7-2. Coin test for safelighting. **A,** Coin placed on unexposed film under safelight. **B,** Developed film showing outline of coin indicating that safelight intensity is too great and not safe.

Overhead white light. There are no special requirements for overhead white light other than providing adequate illumination for the size of the room. The switch for this light should be placed in a position inside the darkroom where it will not be accidentally bumped and turned on, exposing films to white light.

Viewing safelight. Most dental offices will utilize wet readings for emergencies and working films. In these cases it is convenient to have a viewing safelight mounted on the wall behind the processing tanks. In this manner the films can be removed from the fixer after 3 minutes and checked by safelight if they have cleared enough for washing and reading. If a viewing safelight is not located behind the processing tanks, then one would have to hold the wet film up to the overhead safelight with the obvious problem of dripping and staining of the fixer solution. Clearance or the lack of murkiness on the fixed film should never be checked for by holding the film to the overhead white light or the viewbox; in the uncleared state the film can still be affected by the white light.

X-ray viewbox. It is a great convenience to be able to read the wet films in the darkroom. A proper diagnosis can only be made by having an adequate viewing mechanism. The darkroom should have a viewbox to suit these needs. A diagnosis should not be made by holding a wet radiograph up to the overhead light.

Outside warning light. This light should be wired so that when the safelight is on in the darkroom, the warning light is on outside the darkroom. This is a double check on the inside lock on the door and helps to prevent entry into the darkroom when safelight precautions are in effect.

Plumbing

The darkroom requires intake lines of hot and cold water with an adequate drainage line. There should be a thermostatically controlled intake valve in order to maintain constant temperatures of the solutions. The disposal line should be made of materials that will resist the action of the processing chemicals. If automatic processors are going to be used, the rate of flow of the incoming water should be considered. Automatic processors that have continual washing replenishment have requirements in the rate of water flow expressed in gallons per minute. If automatic processing is to be used it should be considered in planning darkroom plumbing.

It is extremely convenient for tank cleaning and solution changing to have a sink with a gooseneck faucet in the darkroom. This is often overlooked in darkroom planning and one will not be reminded of this until the first time the processing tanks have to be carried to the nearest sink for cleaning and replenishing. The gooseneck faucet is essential because a normal size faucet neck will not allow enough room to place the tanks under the faucet for cleaning.

Contents

Processing tanks. Most dental offices have processing units that contain either 1 or 2 gallon developer and fixer inserts suspended in a tank of running water (Fig. 7-3). The tanks should be made of stainless steel and the water bath should have a thermostatically controlled flow valve to keep the solutions at the desired temperature.

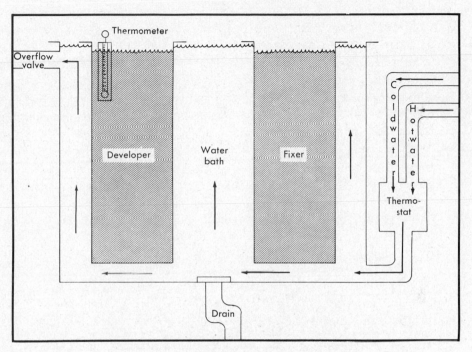

Fig. 7-3. Typical processing tanks in dental office.

Solutions. The developer and fixing solutions are prepared from either the powder or the liquid concentrate, following the manufacturer's directions. Different mixing paddles should be used for the developer and the fixer to prevent cross contamination. Extra amounts of mixed solutions should be stored in dark bottles away from heat and light sources.

Developer and fixing solutions should be changed at least every 3 or 4 weeks. The chemical solutions lose strength when exposed to air and should be replaced regardless of usage factors. If we consider the development of film a chemical reaction, we see that every time the developer and fixer solutions affect a film emulsion the solutions become weakened. In a busy office, it may be necessary to change solutions more frequently than every 3 weeks. Weak developer and fixing solutions will not bring out the optimum image on the film.

Replenisher solutions of developer and fixer are available to compensate for the loss of solutions with use. The replenisher is added in the respective tanks directly to the existing solutions to bring them to the proper fluid level. The level of the solutions should always be kept at the top of the tank to ensure that all immersed films are totally covered with solution. Water should never be added to the solutions to bring them to the desired level; this dilutes the strength of the chemicals. A replenisher should be used or the tank solutions changed completely.

The following chart lists the main ingredients of developer and fixer and their function:

Ingredient	Function
Developer	
Elon or Metol and hydroquinone	Reduces the energized silver bromide crystals to silver
Sodium sulfite	Prevents oxidation of developer
Sodium carbonate	Provides alkaline medium and softens gelatin to allow developing agents to reach silver bromide crystals
Potassium bromide	Controls activity of developing agents and prevents chemical fog
Fixer	
Sodium thiosulfate	Removes undeveloped or unexposed silver bromide crystals from the emulsion
Sodium sulfite	Preservative
Potassium aluminum	Shrinks and hardens gelatin
Acetic acid	Maintains acid medium

200

Timer and thermometer. No darkroom is complete without a timing device and a thermometer. The most modern radiographic equipment will not produce optimum results if there is no time and temperature control in the darkroom. There is no other correct way to process films. The timer is used to determine the length of time the films stay in the developer solution. This depends on the temperature of the developer—not the temperature of the water in the surrounding tanks or that of the water entering through the flow valve. To determine temperature of the developer, a thermometer must be suspended in the developer tank. Early in the day, developer solutions may be cold or hot depending on the overnight office temperature. It may take some time for equalization of temperatures between the water tank and the developing tank. That is why the temperature of the developer bath is read, not the temperature of the water entering the surrounding water tank (Fig. 7-4).

A time-temperature chart, similar to the following, appears on every package of developer-fixer solution. These charts may vary slightly from manufacturer to manufacturer.

80° F 2½ minutes in the developer
75° F 3 minutes in the developer
70° F 4 minutes in the developer
68° F 4½ minutes in the developer
60° F 6 minutes in the developer

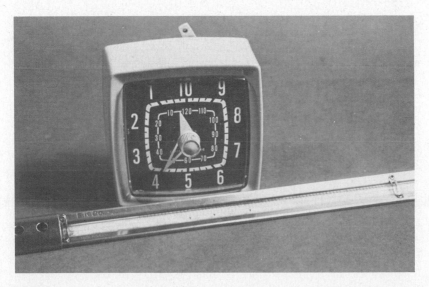

Fig. 7-4. Darkroom timer and thermometer, essential parts of time-temperature technique.

Film hangers. Intraoral film hangers come in various sizes and contain holders for 2 to 20 films. In all cases the films should be unwrapped and attached to the clips without touching the films with one's fingers (Fig. 7-5). This can easily be accomplished by utilizing the wrapping paper in the film packet. The working surface on which the hanger is loaded should be clean and dry to prevent film staining. Film hangers should be numbered or have the patient's name written on the hanger to avoid mixups. The implications of a film series with the wrong patient's name are obvious.

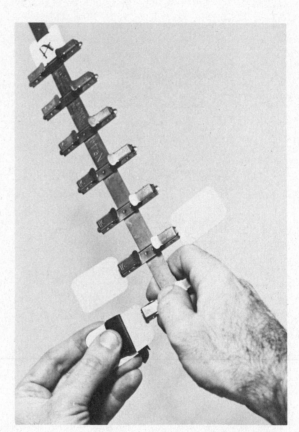

Fig. 7-5. Placing film on hangers in darkroom under safelight conditions. Note that fingers do not touch film.

Dryer. After films have been washed for 20 to 30 minutes they are ready for drying. This can be accomplished by the use of an x-ray dryer or simply by hanging them on towel racks and letting the films air-dry. In either method the films should not touch one another or they will stick together; separating them will rip the emulsion. The drying racks should be out of the way in a clean room. One of the major objections to laboratory-darkroom combinations is that the dust and dirt of the grinding and polishing done in the laboratory will contaminate the dental films.

THE DEVELOPMENT PROCESS

Procedure

1. Lock the darkroom door from the inside and record the patient's names whose films are to be processed on film hangers.
2. Stir the solutions. This is done to equlize the temperature and the chemical distribution of the processing solutions. Use a different stirring paddle for each solution to prevent cross contamination.
3. Check the temperature and set the timer. The temperature of the developer solution should be checked with an accurate thermometer. Refer to the time-temperature chart, which should be posted in the darkroom, and set the time for the desired interval.
4. Turn off the white light and turn on the safelight.
5. Open the film packets and load the film hangers. Work carefully, avoiding finger marks and scratching the film. Be sure the film is securely fastened to film hanger clips.
6. Immerse the film hanger in developer and activate the timer. After immersing the film, immediately raise and lower the hanger a few times so that the film surfaces are totally covered by solution. It is preferable to remain in the darkroom while the films are in the developer. It is permissible to leave if the tank lids are securely in place.
7. Remove the film rack from the developer when the timer sounds.
8. Rinse thoroughly for 20 seconds in the water bath.
9. Place the film rack in the fixer solution. Agitate the rack up and down immediately after the initial placement. Films should remain in the fixer for a minimum of 10 minutes for permanent fixation but may be removed after 3 or 4 minutes for use as a wet reading. After doing this, with the tank lids firmly in place, normal lighting can be resumed in the darkroom. It is not necessary to use safelighting after the timer signals that fixation is completed and films are being moved from the fixer to the water bath.
10. Place the films in the running water bath for 20 minutes.
11. Dry the films. Remove the films from the water bath and suspend them from rack holders to dry.

Latent image

Radiographs, after having been exposed, are said to contain a latent image. The silver bromide on the radiographic emulsion is energized by the x-ray beam. The pattern of this energization of the silver bromide depends on the density of the objects being radiographed. For instance, the silver bromide crystals on the film that lie behind a gold inlay will receive almost no radiation because the dense gold inlay will absorb all the x-ray energy. Silver bromide crystals on the film that correspond to an area such as the pulp of the tooth or a cavity will receive more radiation energy since these areas are less dense and absorb little x-ray energy (Fig. 7-6).

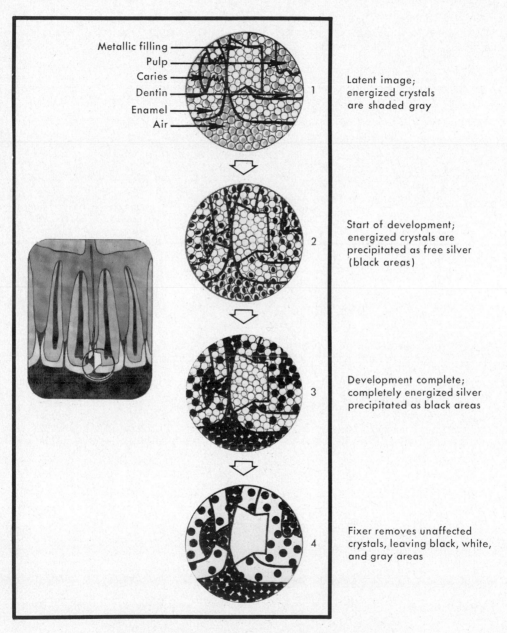

Metallic filling
Pulp
Caries
Dentin
Enamel
Air

1 — Latent image; energized crystals are shaded gray

2 — Start of development; energized crystals are precipitated as free silver (black areas)

3 — Development complete; completely energized silver precipitated as black areas

4 — Fixer removes unaffected crystals, leaving black, white, and gray areas

Fig. 7-6. Schematic drawing of x-ray film development.

Developing

Exposed dental film packets that contain a latent image should be processed as soon as possible. In the darkroom under safelight conditions the x-ray films are removed from the packets and placed on film racks. The developer is the first solution into which these film racks are placed. The developer has a pH above 7 and is basic compared with the acidic fixing solution. The developer chemically reduces the energized silver bromide crystals be precipitating silver on the film base. This precipitation corresponds to the black (radiolucent) areas on the radiograph. An area of less density, such as the pulp, will allow greater penetration of x-rays; therefore, more x-rays will reach that part of the film. The silver bromide crystals will be more greatly energized, and more silver will precipitate to give a black, or radiolucent, outline to the pulp chamber.

This is a chemical reaction. The optimum amount of precipitation of silver for the amount of x-ray energy delivered to the object will take place in a specified amount of time with the developing solution at a certain temperature. This is the basis and importance of the time-temperature technique.

If films are left in the developing solutions too long, more silver will precipitate than was intended and there will be no distinction between dense and less dense structures. A completely overdeveloped film results when all the silver is precipitated by the developer and the film is totally black.

Crystals of silver bromide that have received small amounts of radiation will have correspondingly less silver precipitated and will appear gray. The silver bromide that was unenergized by radiation, such as the area on the film behind a gold crown, will precipitate no silver and will appear white, or radiopaque, on the x-ray film.

Washing (stop-bath)

The main purpose of washing is to remove the developer from the film so that the development process will be stopped. This also removes the basic developer so that it will not contaminate the acidic fixer. This is usually accomplished by agitating the film rack in a water bath for about 20 seconds. Safelight conditions must be maintained when transferring the films from the developer to the wash tank and then to the fixing solution.

Fixing

The acidic fixing solution removes the unexposed and undeveloped silver bromide crystals from the film emulsion and rehardens the emulsion, which has softened during the development process. For permanent fixation the film is kept in the fixing solution for a minimum of 10 minutes. However, films may be removed from the fixing solution after 3 minutes for viewing. This procedure is known as the *wet reading* and is useful when films are needed immediately. For example, a wet reading of a film would be used to check that all the root tip has been removed in an extraction before dismissing the patient.

If these films are to be made part of the patient's permanent record, they should be returned to the fixing solution to complete the required 10 minutes. If this is not done the films will fade and turn brown in a short time.

Washing and drying

The film is washed for about 20 minutes in the water tank to remove the fixing solution from the emulsion. The film is then dried in a clean, dust-free area.

TIME-TEMPERATURE VS SIGHT DEVELOPMENT

The only correct way to process dental x-ray films is by the time-temperature method described in this chapter. It is the scientific method whereby the optimum information is portrayed on the film. In spite of this there are still many dental offices that develop x-ray films by sight. The usual technique is to immerse the film hanger in the developer, removing it at frequent intervals to hold it up to the safelight, until fillings or root shapes are visible. At that point, the films are cleared and placed in the fixer. This is obviously a very inexact, unacceptable technique. The usual reason given for the use of the sight development method is, "We have always done it this way and it works well." This continual acceptance of lower standards of the quality of radiographs leads dentists and dental auxiliaries to believe that this is the way the radiograph should appear. Sight development is unfair to the patient because it does not provide the maximum amount of diagnostic information for the radiation exposure. To repeat, the time-temperature method, done either manually or by automatic processors, is the only acceptable way to process dental radiographs.

RAPID PROCESSING

Rapid processing of dental radiographs is done with either the use of higher solution temperatures, concentrated solutions, agitation of the film, or a combination of these factors. It is sometimes called "hot processing" referring to the temperature of the solutions. Rapid processing can be done with no increase in radiation to the patient but the images produced by this technique are not comparable in density and definition to films processed by the standard methods.

The use of regular strength developing solutions at 92° F with agitation of the film can produce acceptable diagnostic images in less than 1 minute (20 seconds developing, 3 seconds washing, and 30 seconds fixing). There are also concentrated processing solutions available that can be used at room temperature. The increased chemical activity of these solutions makes the rapid processing possible. Some of these solutions use a two bath technique, developer and fixer; others use a single bath technique, or monobath, that contains the developer and the fixer.

207

Rapid processing can be a very helpful technique with endodontic working films and postoperative films in oral surgery where a high degree of definition is not essential. It should not be used for routine processing of films.

EXTRAORAL AND PANORAMIC FILMS

These films are processed in the same manner as intraoral films using the time-temperature technique with the same solutions. The only precaution that must be taken is to check the intensity of the safelight. Those extraoral films that are used in combination with intensifying screens (screen films) are more sensitive to light than nonscreen films. Darkroom illumination that may be safe for intraoral films may adversely affect screen film. The safety of the light can be checked by using the coin test discussed earlier.

CARE AND MAINTENANCE OF THE DARKROOM

Although the maintenance of a darkroom may seem like a housekeeping chore, it is really a means of assuring quality control in the darkroom. Maintenance should be likened to the nurse's regard for sterility to avoid contamination and subsequent infection. Contaminants in the darkroom or other errors due to sloppy techniques may ruin diagnostic radiographs and require retaking of films with an unnecessary increase in the patient's radiation burden.

Cleanliness

The working surface, where films are stripped and placed on hangers, should always be clean and dry. Developer, fixer, and water are the most common stains. Drying films should not be placed above the working surface without catch pans. If the working surface is made of formica, it can easily be cleaned with a mild detergent. Film hangers should be clean and dry when loading films. Hangers used for wet readings are the most likely ones to be insufficiently washed and contain residual fixer that will stain new films.

Processing tanks should be cleaned thoroughly when solutions are changed. This not only means the insert tanks that hold the developer and fixer but also the water reservoir. The water tank will accumulate sludge and algae especially under the metallic lip and in the overflow tube. A bland detergent can be used or, preferably, one of the tank cleaners made specifically for this purpose. It is in this routine cleaning of the tanks that one appreciates the sink and gooseneck faucet in the darkroom.

Hangers

The films should be firmly attached to the hangers so that they will not fall off in the solutions and be lost. As previously mentioned, films should not be fingered but held by the wrapping packets when attaching them to the film clips (see Fig. 7-5).

The film hangers should carefully be placed in and removed from colutions to avoid scratching the emulsions. Hangers with defective clips should be discarded because the defective clip can scratch films on adjacent hangers in the solutions. Defective clips also lead to lost film in the solutions. The idea that the dental auxiliary will remember which clip is defective and avoid using it is not realistic. If the film hanger is in any way defective, it should be discarded.

Hangers should be placed in racks to dry so that films on adjacent hangers do not overlap. If overlapping does occur they will adhere to each other and in separating them the emulsion will tear from the films.

Solutions

Solutions should be brought to the optimal temperature at the beginning of the working day and kept at that temperature by the thermostatic control on the mixing valve.

Tanks should be kept full by the use of replenishers, not by adding water, which dilutes the concentration and weakens the solutions. If the tanks are not kept full, the films or portions of the films on the top clips of the flim rack may not be fully immersed in solution and will not be developed.

Both the developer and fixer solutions should be changed at least every 3 or 4 weeks regardless of use. In some practices with heavy film volume it may be necessary to change solutions as often as once a week.

The lids of the processing tanks should always be closed when the tanks are not in use to prevent oxidation and weakening of the solutions.

Record keeping

Two types of records are important in the darkroom. The first is the supply inventory, including the date of the next scheduled solution change. It is helpful to have the date of the next scheduled solution change posted in a prominent place.

Film identifications are the second type of records that are important in the darkroom; accurate records are essential when processing radiographs. The patient's name, the number of films, the number or letter of the rack the films were placed on, and the date should be recorded. This will eliminate the likelihood of lost films and mixed x-ray series.

Silver retrieval

There are two sources of silver retrieval in the dental office—the old and no longer needed or unusable processed radiographs and the exhausted fixer solution.

Silver can be recovered from the processed radiographs by ashing the film above the melting point of silver. The economic benefit of this endeavor is limited—a pound of radiographs is worth about $30.00.

Residual silver can be retrieved from the fixer by either chemical precipitation or electrolysis. There is no residual silver in the developer solution.

Electrolysis units that can be inserted into dental processing tanks can be purchased for under $100.00. At the present fluctuating price silver retrieval is economically feasible (Fig. 7-7).

The lead foil inserts of film packets can be saved and sold for scrap. Since the foil is very thin, it will take a great amount of it to accumulate a salvageable lot.

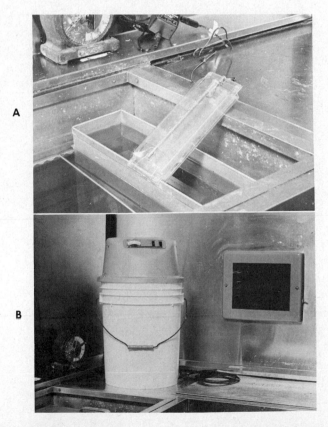

A

B

Fig. 7-7. Silver retrieval units. **A,** Individual office unit. **B,** Large clinic or hospital unit.

QUALITY CONTROL

Quality control testing should be an important part of darkroom maintenance. Periodic checks should be made for light leaks, proper safelighting, and condition of film hangers, accuracy of the thermometer and timer, and the strength of the processing solutions between scheduled changes. It is the chemical strength of the processing solutions that is the greatest variable and daily checks should be done.

The most practical, although admittedly a rough estimate, way to check developer strength in an office is by comparison to a standard. A processed film of ideal density of an average patient should be kept on the darkroom viewbox for comparison of densities. A lessening of density in the processed films would indicate a weakened developer solution.

The strength of the fixer can be gauged by noting the length of time needed to clear films. Fresh, full strength fixer will clear films in 2 to 3 minutes. If clearing requires over 4 minutes, the fixing solution is weakened and should be changed.

AUTOMATIC PROCESSING

In recent years, automatic dental x-ray film processing units have become available. They are not an essential component of a darkroom but a substitute for manual time-temperature processing. Their major advantage is the maintenance of standardized procedure; these units provide solutions of proper strength, correct temperature, and regulated processing time. In short, they provide automated time-temperature processing. Other advantages of the units are the time saved and the increased volume of films that can be processed when compared to the manual method.

The processors vary in the size film they will accept, from only the periapical size to 8- × 10-inch and panoramic films. Some units must be attached to existing plumbing, but others are self-contained. In some safelight procedures are necessary for stripping the film packets and insertion of the film, and others have daylight loaders with light-tight baffles where the hands are placed while inserting the film (Figs. 7-8 and 7-9).

The units contain a series of rollers that carry the film from solution to solution and finally through the drying chamber. A dry film emerges in 5 to 7 minutes.

The machines need periodic cleaning and solution changes and are only as good as the care given them by their operators.

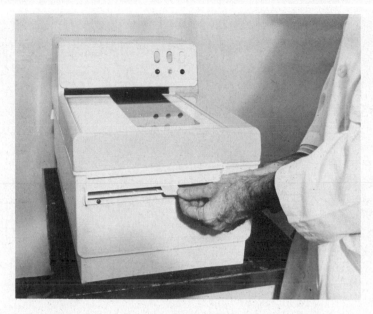

Fig. 7-8. Automatic processor being used in darkroom under safelight conditions.

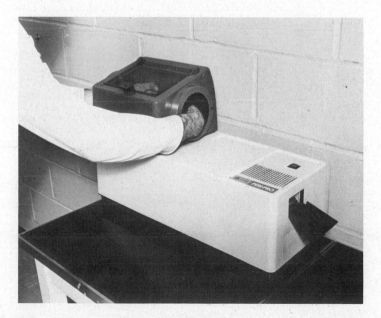

Fig. 7-9. Automatic processor with daylight loader being used in operatory.

DUPLICATING RADIOGRAPHS

In recent years with the increase in dental insurance programs and a more mobile patient population, there are many occasions when it may be necessary to provide radiographs to insurance carriers or forward films to the patient's new dentist. Coupled with this has been the increase in the number of dental malpractice suits where the defendant-dentist's records are of utmost importance. Radiographs are an essential part, if not the most important, of these records. The use of radiographic duplicating film can satisfy requests for radiographs and still maintain the integrity of office records.

Duplicating radiographs is a relatively easy process that requires only a few additions to normal darkroom equipment, namely: duplicating film, 8- × 10-inch film racks, a light source, and a photographic printing frame (Fig. 7-10).

Radiographic duplicating film is readily available from dental supply houses and is supplied in 8- × 10-inch sheets. The photographic emulsion is coated on only one side of the film. Under safelight conditions that emulsion side will appear dull when compared to the shiny, nonemulsion side. The duplicating film is a direct positive film; therefore if more film density is required (darker film) the exposure time is shortened. Conversely, if decreased film density is desired (lighter film) the exposure time is increased. This is just the opposite in time requirements for exposing dental films to x-rays.

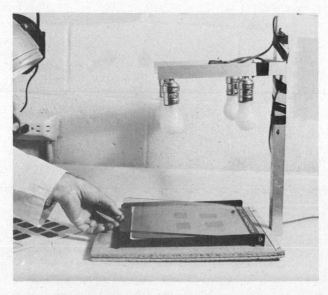

Fig. 7-10. Setup for radiographic duplication.

Procedure

Under safelight conditions, the radiographs to be duplicated are placed in close contact with the emulsion side of the duplicating film. A photographic printing frame is ideal for this because it has a rigid frame with a glass front that will hold the original radiograph against the duplicating film. This frame is placed on a tabletop and exposed to a light source for 4 to 5 seconds with the light source about 2 feet from the film. Since intensities of light sources may vary from office to office, trial exposure should be made to standardize time and light source distance. After the exposure is made, the duplicating film is processed on an 8- × 10-inch film rack in the usual manner. There is no limit to the number of times an original radiograph can be copied. Close positive contact between the radiograph and the duplicating film is essential or a blurred image will occur. The glass top of the printing frame should provide this contact. Films should always be removed from the mounts.

COMMON DARKROOM ERRORS

The following are the most common errors made in the darkroom.

Fogged film (Fig. 7-11)

Fogged film will have an overall gray appearance because of diminished contrast. This can be caused by light leaks in the darkroom or improper safelighting.

Remedy. Test safelight conditions with a coin (see p. 196). Check all doors for possible leaks.

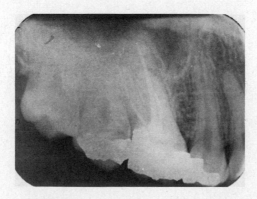

Fig. 7-11. Maxillary molar radiograph that has been fogged. Note lack of definition and contrast.

Underdeveloped film (Fig. 7-12)

Underdeveloped film will be light in appearance and will not contain all the diagnostic information that is possible. This results when the optimum amount of silver has not been precipitated because of weak developing solutions, insufficient developing time, or developing solutions that are too cold.

Remedy. Change the developer and fixing solutions every 3 to 4 weeks and always use the time-temperature method. That is, check the temperature of the developer before immersing the films in the solution and set the timer for the appropriate time as given in the manufacturer's specifications. Refer to density comparison standard mounted on the viewbox to check solution strength.

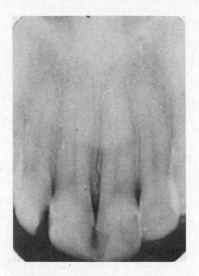

Fig. 7-12. Underdeveloped film.

Overdeveloped film (Fig. 7-13)

Overdeveloped film may vary from dark to totally black, depending on the degree of overdevelopment. This type of film is of no diagnostic value. It results when too much silver has been precipitated on the film base, and in the case of the totally black film, all the silver from the silver bromide has been precipitated. This error can be caused by hot developing solutions or prolonged developing time.

Remedy. Always use the time-temperature method for processing. Be sure that the timer being used has a bell or buzzer that will ring when the developing time has elapsed. This will enable the dental auxiliary to leave the darkroom while the films are being processed. Without the bell the dental auxiliary may be distracted to other duties and forget to remove the films from the developer at the proper time.

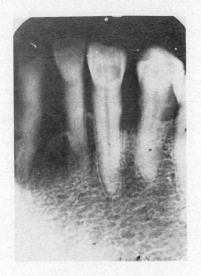

Fig. 7-13. Overdeveloped film.

Developer cutoff (Fig. 7-14)

Cutoff film will show a straight radiopaque border on what was the upper edge of the top film on the processing rack. Actually, this represents an undeveloped area of the film. When the solutions are allowed to deplete in the processing tanks, the films on the top positions on the racks may not be covered by solution when the racks are placed in the tanks. This error should be differentiated from cone cutting, which will give a curved radiopaque border. In cone cutting, the film portion is unexposed; in developer cutoff, the film portion is undeveloped.

Remedy. Always check to see that the processing tanks are full. If the level of solutions has dropped, do not add water. This will only dilute the solution and result in underdeveloped films. Add the proper replenisher solutions to maintain the desired level.

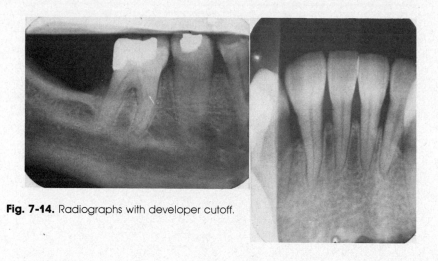

Fig. 7-14. Radiographs with developer cutoff.

Clear films (Fig. 7-15)

Films are clear because the entire emulsion has been washed off. This occurs when films that have had complete fixation are left in running water baths for 24 to 48 hours. This type of film is identical to an unexposed film that is developed and processed. Here the fixer removes all the unaffected silver bromide crystals.

Remedy. Never leave films in water baths overnight. Processing should be complete before you leave the office. Do not leave films in the fixer overnight or for prolonged periods beyond the recommended 10 minutes. The fixer will remove the image.

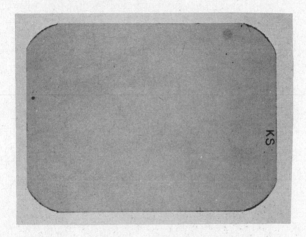

Fig. 7-15. Clear film. This can result from excessive washing or fixing of unexposed film.

Stained films (Fig. 7-16)

If the working surface in the darkroom is wet and dirty, films can be stained either before or after possessing. There is no excuse for this error.

Remedy. Be sure that darkroom work surfaces are kept clean and dry.

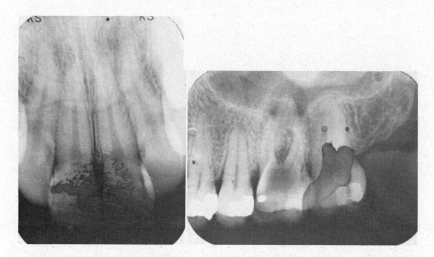

Fig. 7-16. Stained radiograph.

Brown films

Films that have not had adequate fixation (approximately twice the developing time) will turn brown after a period of time and will be useless as part of the patient's permanent record.

Remedy. Make sure all films have adequate fixation time (10 minutes). Return all wet readings to the fixation tank after the patient has been treated.

Torn emulsion (Fig. 7-17)

If films that are drying are allowed to touch and overlap, they will stick together. In separating the films the emulsions are usually torn off the film base in the overlapped area, rendering the film nondiagnostic.

Remedy. Check film racks to be sure that drying films from different racks are not touching.

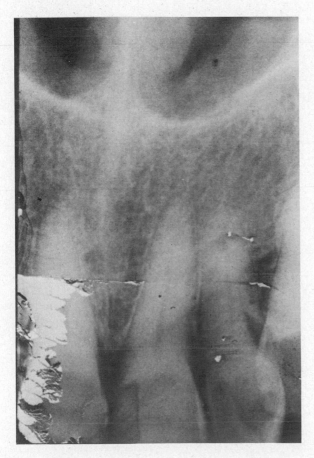

Fig. 7-17. Radiograph with torn emulsion.

Scratched films (Fig. 7-18)

A radiopaque line on a film is usually an artifact caused by scratching the emulsion on the film base in the processing of films. Most often it is caused by putting a second film rack into a tank that already contains a film rack. It can also be caused by fingernails scratching the film while unpacking the film and placing it on a rack.

Remedy. Be careful when putting film racks into the processing solution to avoid touching those already immersed. Discard any film racks that have sharp edges or broken clips that could scratch other films.

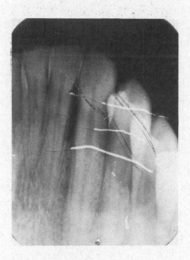

Fig. 7-18. Scratched radiograph.

Lost films in tanks

If films are not firmly clipped onto the racks, they may fall off in any of the three processing baths. A lost film necessitates a retake or results in a wet elbow in an attempt to retrieve it from the processing solution.

Remedy. Check all films to see that they are clipped securely to the rack before processing.

Fluoride artifacts (Fig. 7-19)

Some fluorides, especially stannous fluoride, will produce black marks on radiographs.

Remedy. After working with fluoride, wash hands thoroughly with soap and a weak acid, such as vinegar or lemon juice, before handling films in the darkroom.

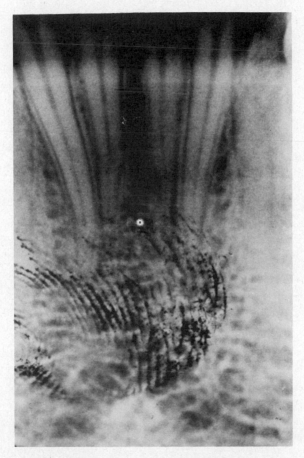

Fig. 7-19. Fluoride artifact. Operator's fingertip contaminated by fluoride touched film when stripping and placing film on hanger.

Reticulation (Fig. 7-20)

If developing is done at an elevated temperature and then the film is placed in a cold water bath, the sudden change in temperature will cause the swollen emulsion to shrink rapidly and give the image a wrinkled appearance called reticulation.

Remedy. Avoid sharp contrasts in temperatures between processing solutions and the water bath.

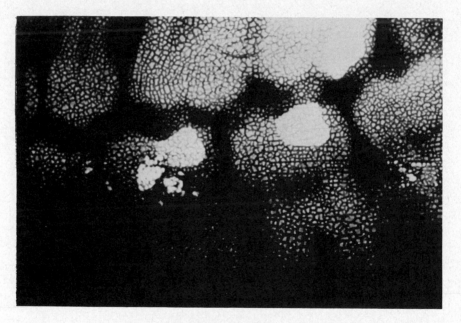

Fig. 7-20. Reticulation.

Air bubbles (Fig. 7-21)

If air bubbles are trapped on the film as it is placed in the processing solutions the chemicals will be prevented from affecting the emulsion in that area.

Remedy. Always agitate the film hangers when placing them in the processing solutions to dislodge any trapped air bubbles.

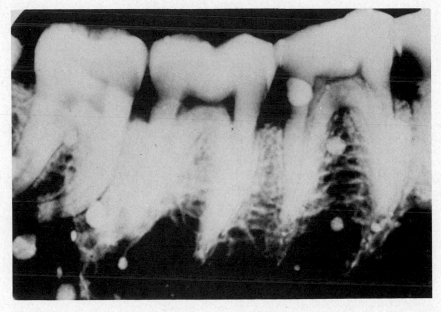

Fig. 7-21. Artifact caused by air bubbles trapped on the film preventing processing solution from touching film in the area.

Static marks (Fig. 7-22)

Static electricity can be produced when intraoral film packets are forcefully opened in the darkroom. The static electricity will produce multiple black linear streaks on the radiograph. The same effect occurs much more frequently on extraoral films. With these films it may happen when removing the piece of film from a full box—the sliding of the film out of the tightly packed box may produce the static electricity. It also may be produced when loading and unloading flexible cassettes in panoramic machines as the film is slid in or out between the intensifying screens. Static electricity may also be created by the dental auxiliary walking around a carpeted office. If the auxiliary does not touch a conductive object before unwrapping the film, the charge marks may result. Static electricity is seen most often on cold, dry days.

Remedy. Ground yourself by touching any conductive object in the darkroom before handling film and avoid friction of any kind against the film that will produce static electricity.

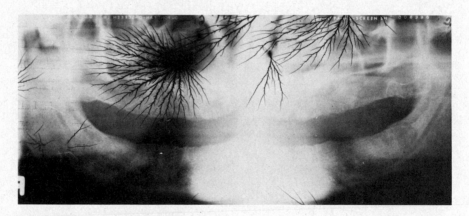

Fig. 7-22. Radiograph with static marks.

Daylight loaders — light leaks (Fig. 7-23)

Film fog, a ruined film, or unusual artifacts can be caused by removing one's hands from the baffle (see Fig. 7-9) before the film has completely entered the processor.

Remedy. Keep your hands on the film until it has been completely taken up by the rollers. The material that makes up the baffle should fit tightly around the hands. Rips and tears should be repaired immediately and stretched elastic replaced. It is a good idea to remove wristwatches and bracelets, because they tend to tear the baffle material.

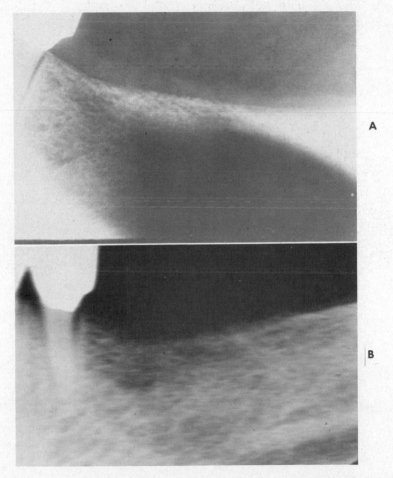

A

B

Fig. 7-23. A, Artifact caused by light leak in daylight loader resembling a large pathologic area in bone. **B,** Normal radiograph of same area.

227

STUDY QUESTIONS

1. List the steps in the processing of dental x-ray film and the purpose of each.
2. What is a safelight? How do you test for reliability?
3. What is the time-temperature technique?
4. List the chemicals that make up the developer and fixer solutions and the function of each.
5. What are the clinical indications for rapid processing? What are its disadvantages?
6. When must safelight conditions be maintained in the darkroom?
7. What are the dental auxiliary's responsibilities in the darkroom?
8. Distinguish between cone cutting and developer cutoff.
9. Can one distinguish between an overexposed film and an overdeveloped film? How?
10. What can cause a clear film?

REFERENCES

1. Biedeman, R.W., and others: A study to develop a rating system and evaluate dental radiographs submitted to a third party carrier, J. Am. Dent. Assoc. **89**:1010, November 1975.

2. Bureau of Radiologic Health: Nashville dental project: an educational approach for voluntary improvement of radiographic health, Rockville, Md., July 1975.

chapter 8 Film mounting and normal radiographic anatomy

The mounting of processed dental radiographs is another important function of the dental auxiliary. It is much easier to view and diagnose radiographs when the films are placed in mounts in their proper anatomic orientation than it is to look at them on a film hanger or sort them from an envelope. Properly mounted films make charting and examination a much more orderly procedure. The mounted films are kept with the patient's chart, and at each subsequent visit the radiographs are place on the viewbox for the dentist to refer to.

Radiographs are identified and oriented as to position in the mouth by the tooth and bony structures visible on each film. A thorough understanding of radiographic anatomy will make mounting an interesting and challenging procedure and not one that is done automatically. Mistakes are made when there is no basic understanding and work becomes tedious and boring.

DESCRIPTIVE TERMINOLOGY

Since we will now be dealing with the processed radiograph in mounting and interpretation, there is a need for certain terms to describe the shades of black, white, and gray that appear. With these terms we can more accurately describe the radiographic findings. The black areas on the radiographs are called *radiolucent* and the white areas are called *radiopaque*. All structures will be either radiolucent or radiopaque but there will be gradation in each category. For instance, metallic fillings are more radiopaque than enamel but both are still radiopaque. Whether a structure appears radiolucent or radiopaque is determined by its object density.

One should never refer to a radiograph as an x-ray. One may say x-ray film but the term x-ray should be used only when referring to the beam of energy that is aimed at the film packet in the patient's mouth. The film is then processed to produce a radiograph.

MOUNTS

Various types of dental film mounts are available. They are usually made of either a cardboard or a celluloidlike material with the desired number of windows for placement of the radiographs (Fig. 8-1). There are 19 window mounts suitable for the adult full-mouth series or four window mounts for the bite-wing survey (Fig. 8-2). The overall size and shape of the mount are made to fit the various types of viewboxes found in dental offices. The area around the film windows may be either clear or opaque. The opaque mounts are preferred because the light is concentrated behind the radiographs and viewing is easier and more diagnostic. If the number of radiographs taken does not fill the mounts, the unused windows should be covered so as not to allow the light to distract the viewer. The black opaque wrapper from the periapical film packet is ideal for this because it is the correct color and size and is easily attached to the mount.

The patient's name, the date, and the number of films taken must be recorded on each mount.

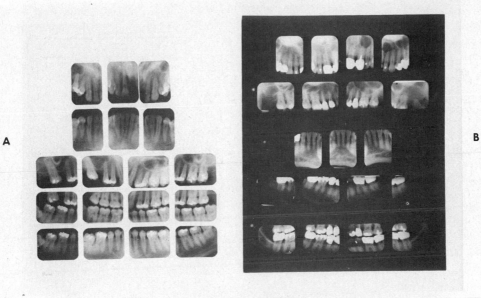

Fig. 8-1. Full-mouth series mounted in **A,** clear celluloid and **B,** opaque mounts.

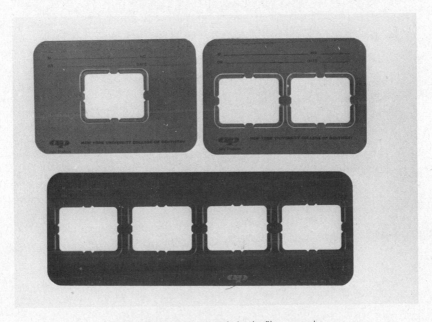

Fig. 8-2. Bite-wing and single film mounts.

MOUNTING

Placement of the radiographs in their correct position in the mounts may seem baffling at first, but if one develops a system based on understanding this problem will be mastered in a short time. One must always work on a light-colored tabletop on which the radiographs can easily be seen when they are laid out. The radiographs are viewed in an illuminator or viewbox placed on the surface where the mounting is being done.

Every radiograph has an embossed or raised dot to help indicate the film orientation. The film packet is placed in the patient's mouth so that the side with the dot is always nearest the occlusal surface of the teeth (see Chapter 3). The film is positioned in the packet by the manufacturer so that the raised portion of the dot faces the x-ray machine when the exposure is made. If you mount the radiographs so that the raised portion of the dot is toward you, you are looking at the film as if you were facing the patient; the patient's left side is on your right (Figs. 8-3 and 8-4). This is called *labial mounting*. If you mount the film so that the depressed side of the dot is toward you, you are looking at the films as if you were viewing them from a position on the patient's tongue; the patient's left side is on your left. This is called *ligual mounting*. Both mounting systems are being used in dentistry today but the trend has been to adopt labial mounting as the universal system.

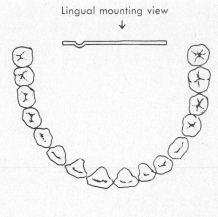

Lingual mounting view
↓

Labial mounting view
↑

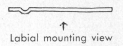

Fig. 8-3. Raised dot on x-ray film and its orientation in film mounts for labial or lingual viewing.

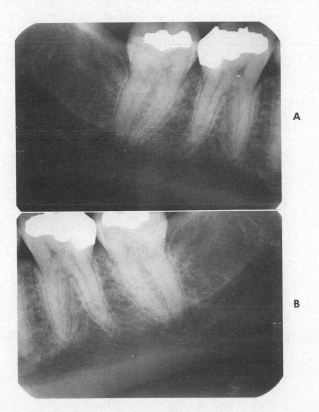

A

B

Fig. 8-4. Same periapical radiograph of right mandibular molar area. **A,** Labial mounting. **B,** Lingual mounting.

233

Procedure

The films from the patient's full-mouth series are laid out on the tabletop and the empty mount placed on the viewbox. The films are placed so that the dots are all one way, either up or down. The films are then divided into three groups: bite-wings, anterior periapicals, and posterior periapicals. The bite-wing films are easily identified because the crowns of both the upper and lower teeth are seen. The anterior and posterior periapical films are differentiated by the vertical orientation on the film for anterior teeth and the horizontal orientation for posterior teeth.

The maxillary anterior films are then differentiated from the mandibular anteriors on the basis of root and crown shape and anatomic landmarks that will be discussed later. The films are then placed in their proper position in the mount. The same routine is repeated for the posterior films. The bite-wing films are mounted last. Since they show only the crowns of the teeth there are no root shapes and surrounding bony landmarks to aid in anatomic identification. Once the periapicals are mounted, fillings and missing teeth can be used to help identify and orient the bite-wing films.

There are certain generalizations that can be made about crown and root shapes that are seen on radiographs. The following hints will aid the novice in mounting films:

1. Crowns of upper anterior central and lateral incisors are wider than those of lower central and lateral incisors.
2. Maxillary premolars usually have two roots; mandibular premolars have one root.
3. Mandibular first and second molars usually have two divergent curved roots with bone clearly visible between them. This is particularly true of the first molar. Maxillary molars have three roots, two buccal and one palatal. The large palatal root obscures the interradicular bone.

These aids, along with the anatomic landmarks that will be described on the following pages, will enable the dental auxiliary to properly orient radiographs in the x-ray film mount.

NORMAL RADIOGRAPHIC ANATOMY

In order to fully utilize and properly interpret radiographs, the dental auxiliary must be thoroughly familiar with normal radiographic anatomy. This includes all the structures seen on periapical, bite-wing, occlusal, panoramic, and extraoral projections. The first consideration in diagnosing a suspected lesion should be to differentiate it from a normal structure. This may often be difficult because there are wide variations of normal in the gross anatomy in regard to size, shape, and location that may be further modified by age, use, and disuse. Radiographically, these variations may be further exaggerated by the projection and angulation used. All landmarks are not always demonstrable on every full-mouth survey or individual film. When confronted by a suspicious lesion, the first things considered are the anatomic landmarks normally seen in that particular area.

In interpreting radiographic landmarks, it is important that the gross configuration of the structure be kept in mind. A thick bony structure such as a ridge or muscle attachment will appear more radiopaque because of increased object density. Any foramen, cavity, or concavity of bone will produce an area that will be represented on the film as a radiolucency because of decreased density. Radiographs, being two-dimensional representations, will produce superimpositions of many normal structures that can be misleading and this should be kept in mind when interpreting films.

Radiographs are two-dimensional pictures of a three-dimensional object. Radiographs do not portray depth; teeth may be superimposed on anatomic structures in the skull that may be millimeters in front of or in back of them. The best example of this is the roots of the maxillary molars and the maxillary sinus. Very few molar roots are actually in the sinus although they may appear that way on almost all molar radiographs (see Fig. 8-22).

RADIOGRAPHIC TOOTH ANATOMY

The component structures of the tooth and its supporting structures are well defined on the dental radiograph because of their differences in density (Fig. 8-5).

Enamel is the densest and thus the most radiopaque of the natural tooth structures. It is seen as a radiopaque band that covers the crown of the tooth and ends in a fine edge at the cementoenamel junction.

Dentin is the next layer of tooth structure. It is not as highly calcified as enamel and thus not as radiopaque. It comprises the major part of the tooth structure and is seen in both the crown and the root portions.

Cementum is the thin covering on the surface of the root of the tooth. It is difficult to distinguish cementum from dentin because it is thin and its density is not very different from that of dentin. Cementum is best seen in the pathologic condition hypercementosis, which is an overgrowth of cementum.

The *pulp chamber* and the *root canal* are seen as a continuous radiolucent space in the center of the crown and root of the tooth. The fingerlike projections in the coronal portion are called *pulp horns*. They are seen most often in young patients because the pulp chambers of teeth become smaller with age and in some cases may be totally obliterated by secondary dentin.

The *periodontal membrane* is seen as a radiolucent line about 0.5 mm wide between the cementum of the root of the tooth and the lamina dura. The periodontal membrane may not always be seen clearly on every root surface because of differences in horizontal angulation when the radiograph was taken.

The *lamina dura* is a radiopaque line that surrounds the periodontal membrane. It represents the bony wall of the tooth socket. It may not be seen on every surface because of angulation.

The *alveolar bone* is the bone that supports the teeth. It is comprised of cancellous and cortical-compact bone. The cancellous bone is seen as a series of small radiolucent compartments called *medullary spaces*. These spaces are separated by a radiopaque honeycomb called *trabeculae*. The occlusal part of the alveolar bone is referred to as the *alveolar crest*. The mandible is a much denser bone than the maxilla; hence the medullary spaces are smaller and there is greater trabeculation in the mandible.

The *cortical bone* is seen as a dense radiopaque structure that comprises the buccal and palatal plates of the maxilla and the buccal and lingual plates as well as the inferior border of the mandible.

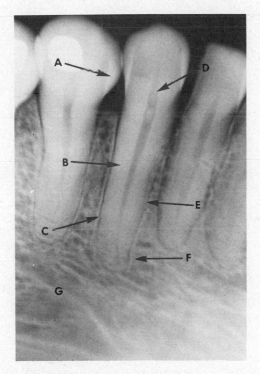

Fig. 8-5. Normal radiographic tooth anatomy: *A*, enamel; *B*, dentin; *C*, periodontal membrane; *D*, pulp chamber; *E*, cementum; *F*, lamina dura; *G*, alveolar bone.

TOOTH DEVELOPMENT

The developing tooth can be seen at all stages on radiographs. The tooth germ (Fig. 8-6) prior to calcification appears as a round or oval radiolucency in the body of the maxilla or mandible. As crown formation progresses the radiolucent follicle is seen surrounding the crown of the tooth (Fig. 8-7). After the tooth erupts the dental papilla can be seen at the forming apices (Fig. 8-8).

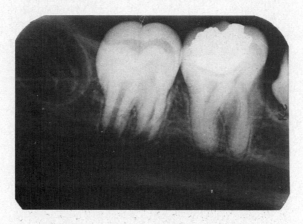

Fig. 8-6. Tooth germ of mandibular third molar.

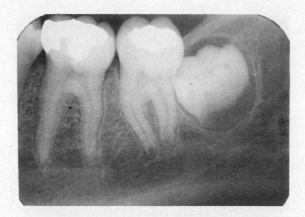

Fig. 8-7. Follicle of mandibular third molar.

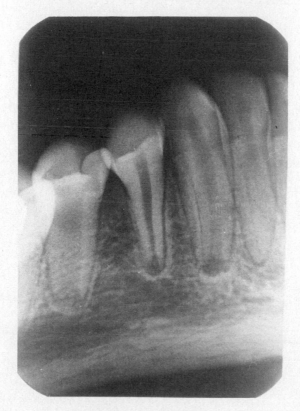

Fig. 8-8. Dental papilla.

Radiographic examination by either the standard full-mouth series or panoramic films is essential in determining the progress and pattern of tooth eruption (Figs. 8-9 and 8-10). In this manner conditions such as premature loss of primary teeth, anodontia, over-retained teeth, ankylosis, tumors, and supernumerary teeth that will affect the eruption pattern can be identified (Figs. 8-11 and 8-12).

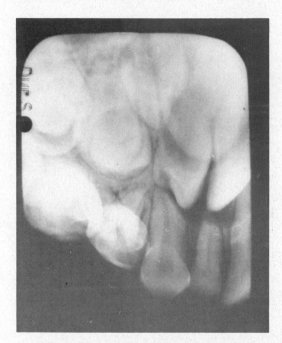

Fig. 8-9. Mixed dentition of child.

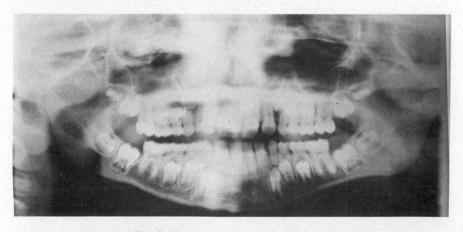

Fig. 8-10. Mixed dentition on panoramic film.

240

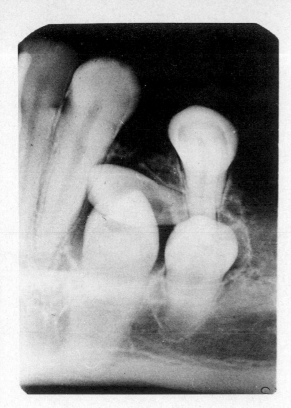

Fig. 8-11. Supernumerary tooth blocking eruption of first premolar.

Fig. 8-12. Tumor (odontoma) blocking eruption of maxillary canine.

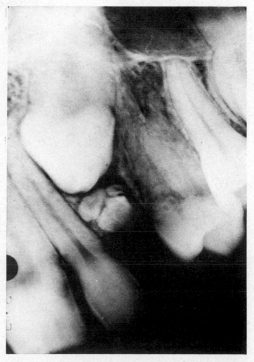

RESTORATIONS

Metallic restorations such as gold inlays, crowns, foils, posts, pins, or silver amalgam are the most radiopaque areas seen on radiographs (Figs. 8-13 and 8-14). One can distinguish between them only on the basis of size and shape, not on the degree of radiopacity. The synthetic restorations used in anterior teeth (such as porcelain, acrylics, and composites) (Fig. 8-15) appear radiolucent and may be mistaken radiographically for caries. Recently manufacturers of some synthetic restorations have incorporated radiopaque particles in their preparations so that the restorations can be distinguished from caries (Fig. 8-16). Temporary or sedative fillings and cavity liners, such as zinc oxide, calcium hydroxide, zinc, oxyphosphate, and cement, appear radiopaque since they contain some metallic elements (see Figs. 8-13 and 8-15). Porcelain jackets will appear slightly radiopaque, with the radiopaque cement being more apparent (see Fig. 8-14, A). Endodontic fillings will appear as radiopaque fillings in the pulp and root canal chambers. Of the two types of endodontic fillings most commonly used, the silver cones will appear more radiopaque than the gutta-percha points (Fig. 8-17). Other materials that can be seen are fractures wires (Fig. 8-18) and orthodontic bands and wires (Fig. 8-19).

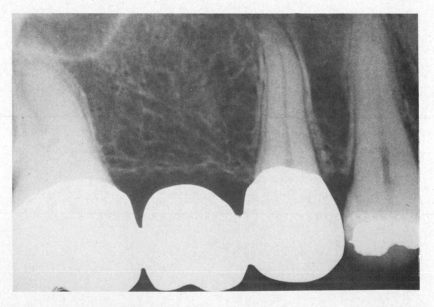

Fig. 8-13. Fixed bridge and amalgam restoration. Note that acrylic facing of pontic does not appear on radiograph. Also note difference in radiopacities between amalgam and its cement base.

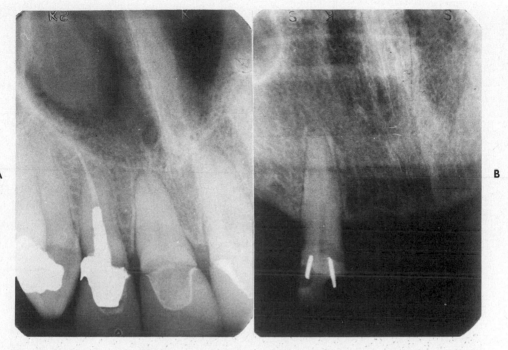

A B

Fig. 8-14. A, Gold post and core under porcelain jacket. **B,** Metallic pins under synthetic restoration.

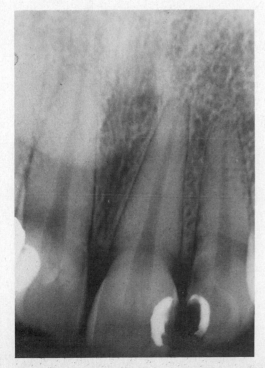

Fig. 8-15. Radiolucent anterior synthetic restorations with cement bases.

243

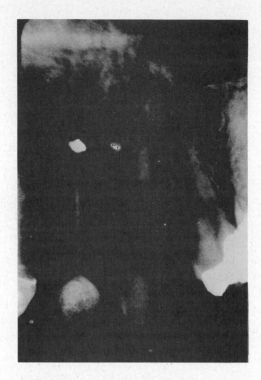

Fig. 8-16. Radiopaque anterior synthetic restorations, lateral incisor and canine. Note radiopaque gutta-percha endodontic filling and retrograde amalgam.

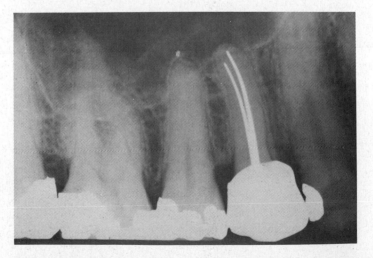

Fig. 8-17. Silver cones used as endodontic filling material in first premolar.

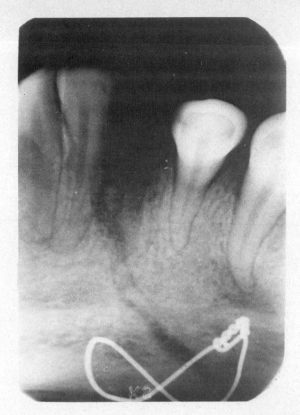

Fig. 8-18. Healing mandibular fracture with intraosseous wires in place.

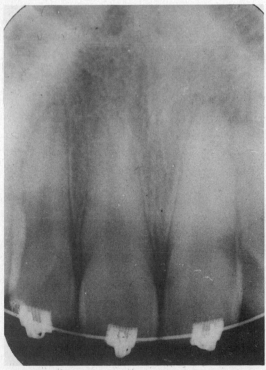

Fig. 8-19. Orthodontic brackets and wires.

RADIOGRAPHIC ANATOMY OF MAXILLA AND MANDIBLE

Maxilla

Maxillary incisor area (Fig, 8-20). The nasopalatine (incisive) foramen is seen as an oval radiolucency between the roots of the maxillary central incisors. In some radiographs the incisive canal can be seen leading to the foramen. The foramen is actually in the anterior portion of the palate, but superimposition makes it appear to be located between the roots of the central incisors. The position of the nasopalatine foramen on the radiograph may vary from just above the crest of the alveolar ridge to the level of the apices of the teeth because of anatomic variations and vertical angulation. In some cases, the shadow of the foramen may be superimposed on the apex of a central incisor and must be differentiated from periapical disease.

The median palatine suture is seen as a thin radiolucent line running vertically between the roots of the maxillary central incisors. It must be differentiated from a fracture line, nutrient canal, and fistulous tract.

The nasal fossa is the paired radiolucent structure that is seen superior to the apices of the incisor teeth. The fossa is also seen on the canine projection where it may overlap or appear to adjoin the maxillary sinus. The radiopaque band that separates the left and right nasal fossa is called the median nasal septum. The septum ends inferiorly in the V shaped radiopaque anterior nasal spine.

The anterior nasal spine may be seen near or superimposed upon the incisive foramen. The radiopacity that is sometimes seen projecting into the fossa from its lateral wall is the inferior concha (turbinate).

The soft tissue and cartilaginous shadow of the tip of the nose as well as the soft tissue outline of the lip may be seen superimposed from the crest of the ridge to the crowns of the teeth. These soft tissue shadows are seen most clearly on edentulous films where even the nares (openings) of the nose as well as the columella (separating column) are seen.

The lateral fossa is a depression in the labial plate in the lateral incisor region. It will appear as a radiolucency between the lateral incisor and canine since it represents an area of thin bone.

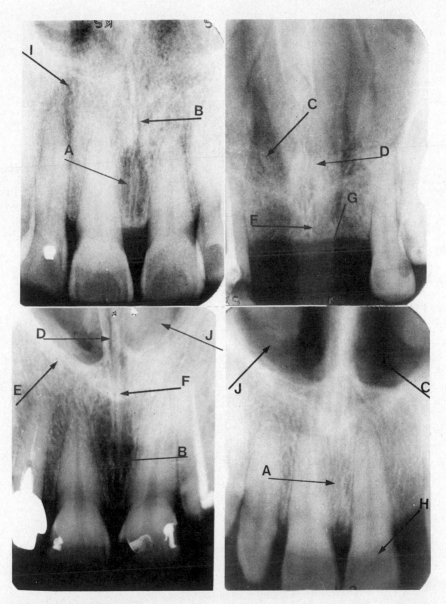

Fig. 8-20. Maxillary central incisor area. *A,* Naso-palatine foramen; *B,* median palatine suture; *C,* nasal fossa; *D,* median nasal septum; *E,* floor of nasal cavity; *F,* anterior nasal spine; *G,* columnella of nose; *H,* lip line; *I,* lateral fossa; *J,* inferior concha.

Maxillary canine area (Fig. 8-21). In the maxillary canine region two large radiolucent areas are seen. The more mesial area is the lateral aspect of the nasal fossa and the more distal aspect is the anterior extent of the maxillary sinus. In the edentulous film, the radiopaque Y formed by the anterior and inferior border of the maxillary sinus as the arms and the floor of the nasal cavity as the stem of the Y are useful in mounting orientation.

The radiopaque shadow of the nose may also be seen on canine area radiographs. In some projections a radiolucent area is seen distal to the canine and represents the nasolabial fold.

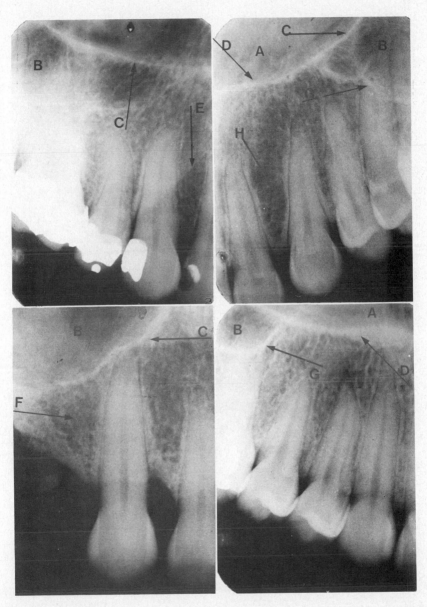

Fig. 8-21. Maxillary canine area. *A,* Nasal fossa; *B,* maxillary sinus; *C,* septum of bone separating maxillary sinus and nasal septum; *D,* floor of nasal cavity; *E,* shadow of the nose; *F,* nasolabial fold; *G,* floor of maxillary sinus; *H,* lateral fossa.

249

Maxillary premolar area (Fig. 8-22). In the maxillary premolar area the radiolucent maxillary sinus may be seen either superimposed on, between, or above the apices of the teeth. It is not always visible since the size and position of the maxillary sinus may vary from patient to patient. The floor of the maxillary sinus is seen as a radiopaque line running horizontally at its lower border. The floor of the nasal fossa may be seen as a radiopaque line running horizontally at the superior portion of the maxillary sinus. Nutrient canals may be seen in the alveolar bone as well as grooves for vessels in the walls of the maxillary sinus. Bony septum may also be seen in the maxillary sinus.

The edentulous premolar radiograph is identified by the presence of the maxillary sinus. It is differentiated from the molar radiograph by the absence of the maxillary sinus in the mesial part of the film and the start of the radiopaque zygomatic arch band at the distal portion of the film.

In some edentulous films the shadow of the buccinator muscle is seen. This shadow makes part of the normally radiolucent area below the ridge appear radiopaque because of the increased density of the muscle.

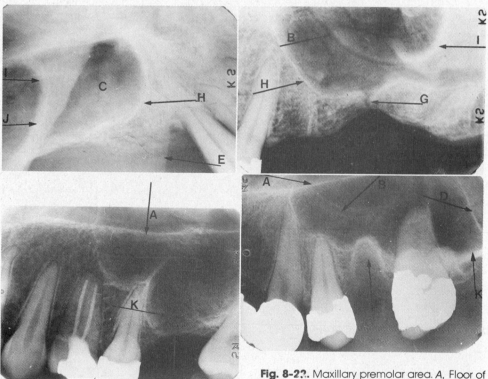

Fig. 8-22. Maxillary premolar area. A, Floor of nasal fossa; B, nutrient canals in sinus wall; C, maxillary sinus; D, sinus septum; E, buccinator shadow; F, extraction socket; G, oral antral communication; H, floor of maxillary sinus; I, zygomatic process of maxilla; J, zygomatic arch; K, pneumatization.

Maxillary molar area (Fig. 8-23). The maxillary sinus is a radiolucent area that is always seen on periapical projections of the maxillary molar region. The sinus may be unilocular or compartmented by bony septa. Radiopaque spurs or ridges may be seen projecting into the sinus and radiolucent tracts or grooves, representing blood vessel positions, may be seen in the walls of the sinus. The size of the maxillary sinus varies greatly because of age, morphology, and the radiographic projection. The sinuses in a patient may be asymmetrical and may tend to enlarge or grow into areas of the alveolar ridge where teeth have been extracted. This process is called *pneumatization*. Just distal to the third molar ridge area is the maxillary tuberosity. This area of cancellous bone may also contain the posterior extension of the maxillary sinus. The large fibrous buildup of soft tissue above the tuberosity may cause a slightly radiopaque shadow on the radiograph and is called the *tuberosity pad*.

The zygomatic process of the maxilla is seen as an inverted U shaped radiopacity superimposed upon the roots of the first and second molars and the maxillary sinus. The malar bone (zygoma), which is a continuation of the zygomatic process, is seen as a broad uniform radiopaque band that extends posteriorly. Together they make up the zygomatic arch.

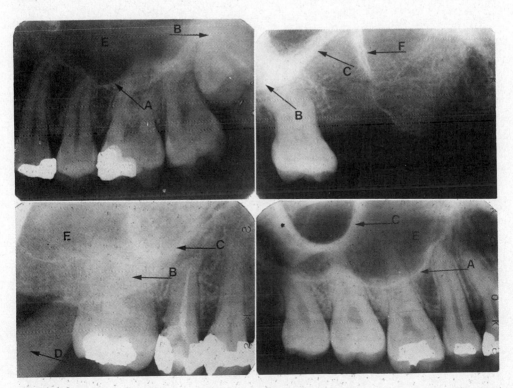

Fig. 8-23. Maxillary molar area. *A,* Floor of sinus; *B,* zygomatic arch; *C,* zygomatic process of maxilla; *D,* coronoid process of mandible; *E,* maxillary sinus; *F,* septum in sinus.

The hamular process is the radiopaque projection that extends downward distal to the posterior surface of the maxillary tuberosity. It is the inferior end of the medial ptery-goid plate of the sphenoid bone. The radiolucent area between the tuberosity and the hamular process is referred to as the hamular notch (Fig. 8-24).

In the distal inferior portion of maxillary molar radiographs a large radiopaque structure may be seen. This is the coronoid process of the mandible. When an edentulous series is mounted this landmark is helpful in determining which is the most distal of the maxillary radiographs.

The maxillary torus is a lobulated bony growth in the midline of the palate. When seen on a periapical radiograph it will appear as a dense, well-demarcated, radiopaque area (Fig. 8-25).

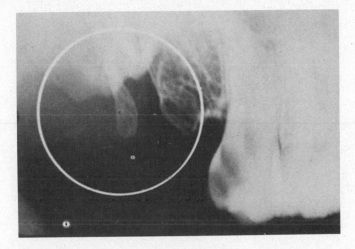

Fig. 8-24. Posterior part of maxillary molar region. In circle are maxillary tuberosity, hamular notch, and hamular process.

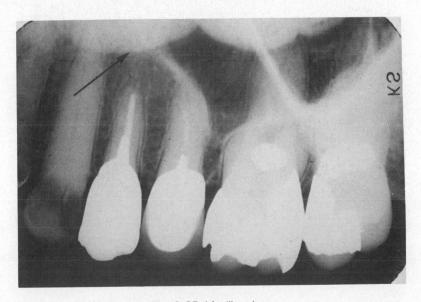

Fig. 8-25. Maxillary torus.

Mandible

Mandibular incisor area (Fig. 8-26). In the mandibular central incisor area, just below the apices of the central incisors in the midline, there is often a somewhat circular radiopacity. This is the genial tubercle, which represents a bony growth on the lingual surface of the mandible to which muscles are attached. In the middle of the genial tubercle a small circular radiolucency may be seen. This is the lingual foramen, which is the exit point from the mandible for the lingual branches of the incisive vessels. Nutrient canals, although found in all areas of the mandible and maxilla, are seen most easily in this area. They appear as radiolucent lines that run vertically in the alveolar bone and terminate in small circular radiolucent nutrient foramina. The nutrient canals are pathways for blood vessels and nerves.

The mental ridge is a broad radiopaque band that represents a ridge of bone on the labial aspect of the mandible. It arises bilaterally below the apical area of the canine and incisors and runs medially and upward toward the mandibular symphysis. The ridge, if superimposed over the apices of the teeth, may hinder diagnosis. The ridge should be differentiated from the internal oblique ridge.

The shadow of the lip is seen on anterior radiographs. That portion of the film not covered by the lip will appear darker than the rest of the film because there is no soft tissue attenuation in the area. The lip line, unless identified as such, can hinder radiographic interpretation.

The inferior border of the mandible is seen as a broad radiopaque band that represents the thick cortical bone of this area.

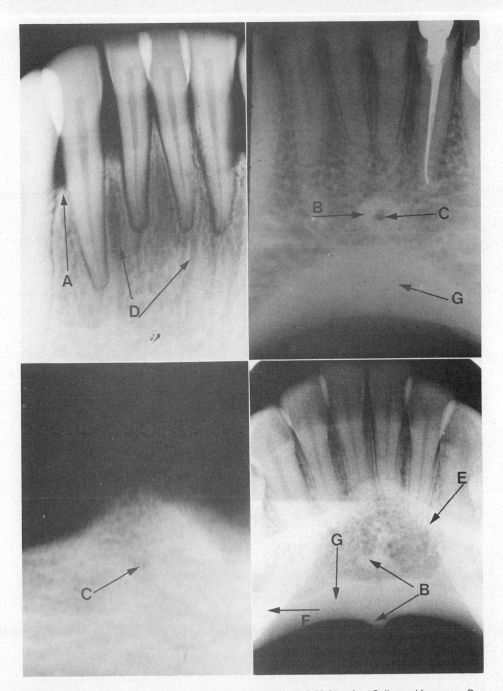

Fig. 8-26. Mandibular incisor area. *A*, Alveolar ridge; *B*, genial tubercles; *C*, lingual foramen; *D*, nutrient canals; *E*, mental ridge; *F*, mylohyoid ridge; *G*, inferior border of mandible.

Mandibular canine area (Fig. 8-27). The anterior extension of the internal oblique ridge and submandibular fossa can be seen in the canine area.

The edentulous mandibular canine may be difficult to orient in the mount. One should look for the genial tubercle on the mesial part of the film and possibly the mental foramen in the distal part. The edentulous alveolar ridge crest will slope downward as it goes distally.

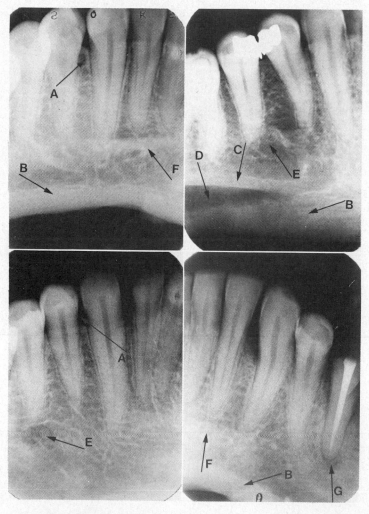

Fig. 8-27. Mandibular canine area. *A,* Alveolar ridge; *B,* inferior border of mandible; *C,* internal oblique ridge; *D,* submandibular fossa; *E,* mental foramen; *F,* mental ridge; *G,* periapical pathology.

256

Mandibular premolar area (Fig. 8-28). The mental foramen is seen as a round or oval radiolucency found near the apices of the premolars. The mental foramen may be found between, below, or even superimposed on the apices of the premolars. It is through this foramen that the mental nerves and blood vessels emerge. In some cases the radiolucent mandibular canal can be seen leading directly to the foramen.

The termination of the external oblique ridge can be seen in this area as well as the internal oblique ridge, submandibular fossa, and inferior border of the mandible.

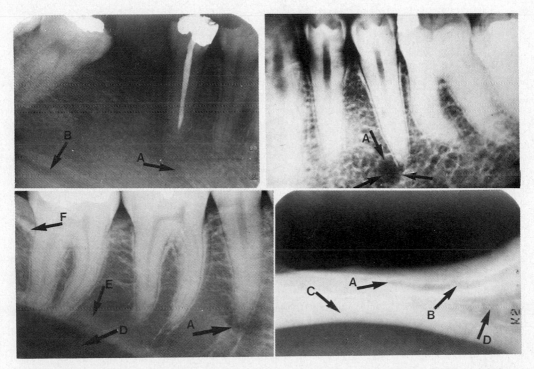

Fig. 8-28. Mandibular premolar area. *A*, Mental foramen; *B*, mandibular canal; *C*, inferior border of the mandible; *D*, submandibular fossa; *E*, internal oblique ridge; *F*, external oblique ridge.

The mandibular tori, although not strictly considered normal landmarks, because of their frequency are included in this section. They are seen singularly or multiply and usually bilaterally on the lingual aspects of the mandible in or near the premolar region. They appear as clearly outlined radiopacities (Fig. 8-29).

The edentulous premolar film is identified and oriented for mounting by the presence of the mental foramen and the ending of the external oblique ridge. The crest of the edentulous alveolar ridge tends to rise as it goes mesially.

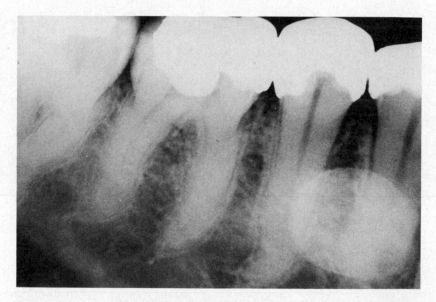

Fig. 8-29. Mandibular tori.

Mandibular molar area (Fig. 8-30). The mandibular canal is seen as a radiolucent band below the apices of the posterior teeth, originating at the mandibular foramen and running downward and forward to end at the mental foramen. It is bordered by thin, radiopaque lines.

The oblique ridges refer to the internal and external oblique ridges. The external ridge, a continuation of the anterior border of the ramus, is seen as a radiopaque line that passes diagonally down and forward across the molar region. The internal or mylohyoid ridge is a radiopaque line that runs from the medial and anterior aspect of the ramus downward and forward to end at the lower border of the symphysis. When these two ridges are seen together the internal oblique ridge is the lower of the two radiopaque lines.

The submandibular fossa is seen as a radiolucent area below the mylohyoid ridge. It represents an area of reduced thickness of bone caused by a depression on the medial surface of the mandible. This radiolucency may be accentuated by a prominent mylohyoid ridge and a thick, opaque, inferior border of the mandible.

Nutrient canals are seen commonly in the molar region especially when it is edentulous.

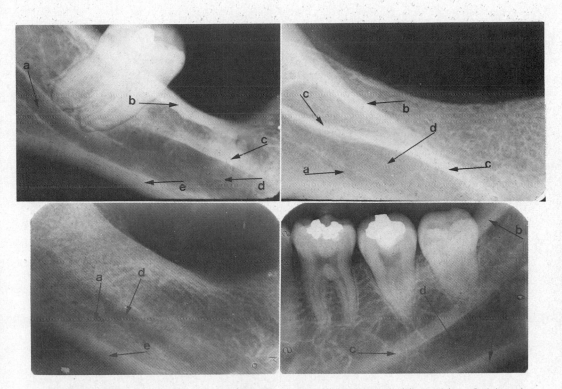

Fig. 8-30. Mandibular molar area. *A,* Mandibular canal; *B,* external oblique ridge; *C,* internal oblique ridge; *D,* submandibular fossa; *E,* inferior border of mandible.

259

RADIOGRAPHIC ANATOMY FOR PANORAMIC FILMS

The normal radiographic anatomy for panoramic films is seen in Fig. 8-31. Some of the anatomic landmarks listed have been described in the preceding section on periapical radiographs. Those landmarks commonly seen on panoramic films that are diagnostically important are also discussed here.

The mandibular foramen. The mandibular foramen appears as an oval radiolucency that is seen at the origin of the mandibular canal at the midpoint of the ramus of the mandible.

The pharyngeal air space. The pharyngeal air space appears as a bilateral symmetrical radiolucent band that is seen between the radiopaque palatal line and the apices of the maxillary posterior teeth. It runs posteriorly and downward across the ramus and into the soft tissues of the neck. The appearance of the air space on radiographs varies depending on the position of the tongue and thus the air above it and the state of contraction of the pharyngeal muscles. The diagnostic key for the air space is the bilateral and symmetrical appearance that can be followed running distally off the bone into the soft tissue.

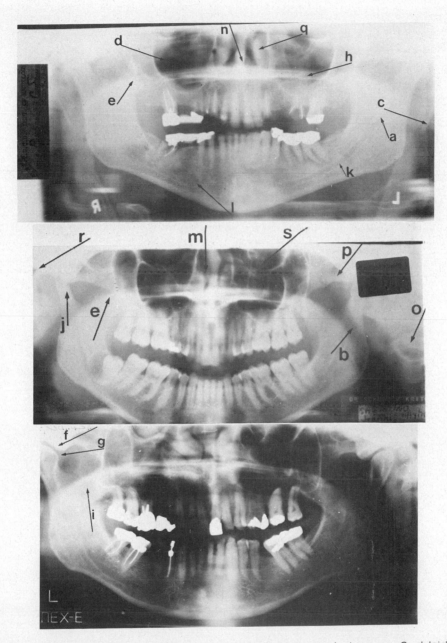

Fig. 8-31. Panoramic film. *A*, Mandibular foramen; *B*, pharyngeal air space; *C*, styloid process; *D*, maxillary sinus; *E*, coronoid process; *F*, articular eminence; *G*, glenoid fossa; *H*, hard palate; *I*, mental foramen; *J*, mandibular condyle; *K*, mandibular canal; *L*, mental foramen; *M*, nasal fossa; *N*, nasal septum; *O*, cervical vertebrae; *P*, zygoma; *Q*, inferior turbinate; *R*, external auditory meatus; *S*, orbit.

The styloid process. The styloid process is a radiopaque projection that may be seen bilaterally projecting downward just posterior to the ramus of the mandible. The styloid ligaments attached to the process may calcify and give the appearance of an abnormally long styloid process. The calcification of the ligament may not be continuous or may start at the attachment of the ligament to the styloid process, giving the appearance of a fracture of the styloid process (Fig. 8-32).

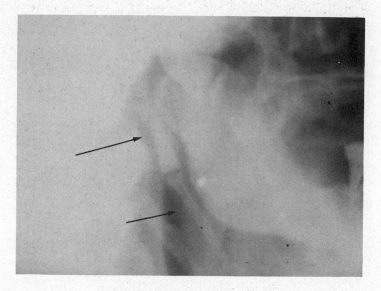

Fig. 8-32. Calcified styloid ligament.

OCCLUSAL PROJECTIONS (Figs. 8-33 and 8-34)

It is important to keep in mind in the interpretation of occlusal films that the projection is in the superoinferior plane and shows the third dimension not seen in periapical, bite-wing, and panoramic films. The type of occlusal projection used, right-angle or topographic (65 degrees), should also be considered because the position of the landmarks will vary depending on angulation.

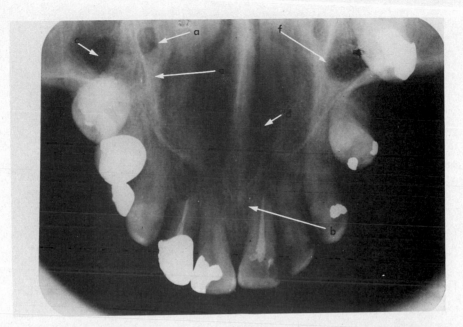

Fig. 8-33. Maxillary occlusal film: *a*, nasolacrimal duct; *b*, anterior palatine foramen; *c*, maxillary sinus; *d*, nasal fossa; *e*, lateral wall of nasal fossa; *f*, lateral wall of maxillary sinus.

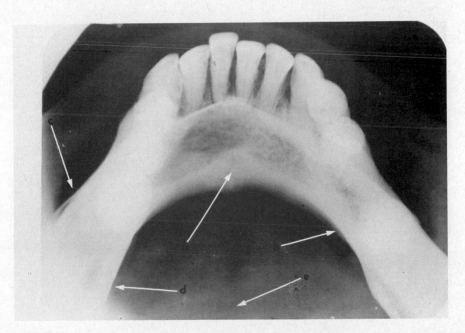

Fig. 8-34. Mandibular occlusal film: *a*, genial tubercles; *b*, inferior border; *c*, buccal cortical plate; *d*, lingual cortical plate; *e*, shadow of tongue.

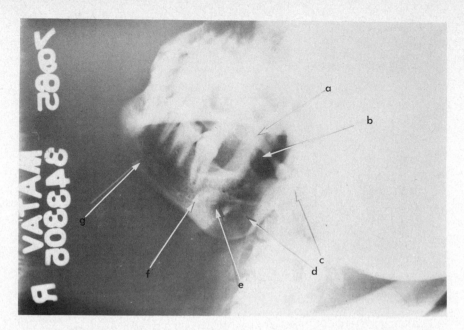

Fig. 8-35. Lateral oblique projection of mandible: *a*, coronoid process; *b*, sigmoid notch; *c*, condyle; *d*, pharyngeal air space; *e*, mandibular foramen; *f*, mandibular canal; *g*, mental foramen.

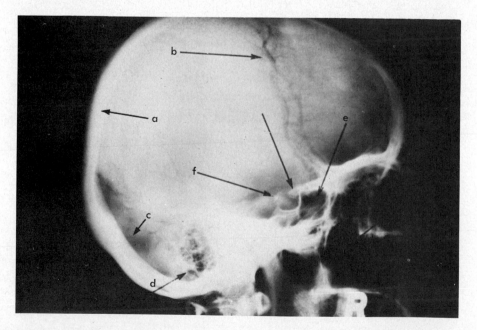

Fig. 8-36. Lateral skull projection: *a*, inner and outer table; *b*, vascular markings; *c*, lateral venous sinus; *d*, mastoid air cells; *e*, sphenoid sinus; *f*, anterior and posterior clinoid processes, sella turcica.

264

EXTRAORAL PROJECTIONS

The most commonly seen and important landmarks for the extraoral techniques described in Chapter 5 are given in Figs. 8-35 to 8-39.

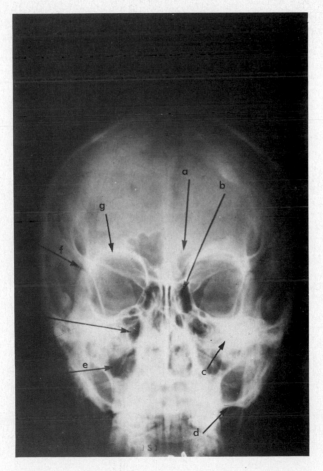

Fig. 8-37. Posteroanterior view: *a*, frontal sinus; *b*, ethmoid sinus; *c*, petrous ridge; *d*, base of skull; *e*, maxillary sinus; *f*, frontozygomatic suture; *g*, orbit.

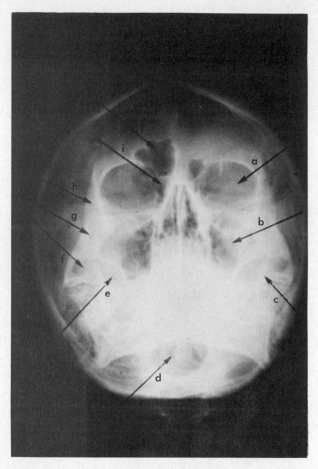

Fig. 8-38. Posteroanterior view of sinuses (Waters' view): *a*, orbit; *b*, maxillary sinus; *c*, coronoid process; *d*, foramen magnum and vertebra; *e*, lateral wall of maxillary sinus; *f*, zygomatic arch; *g*, malar bone; *h*, frontozygomatic suture; *i*, ethmoid sinus; *j*, frontal sinus.

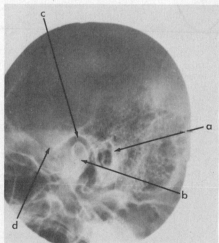

Fig. 8-39. Normal temporomandibular joint: *a*, external auditory meatus; *b*, condyle; *c*, articular fossa; *d*, articular eminence.

266

STUDY QUESTIONS

1. Define radiolucent and radiopaque. Give an example of each.
2. In the labial mounting technique, what is the film orientation in relation to the viewer?
3. Radiographically how could we differentiate the mandibular molar edentulous film from the maxillary molar edentulous film?
4. On what radiographic projection is the coronoid process of the mandible seen?
5. Why is the mental foramen seen as a radiolucency?
6. Which is the most radiopaque of the natural tooth structures? Which is the most radiolucent?
7. On what projections is the maxillary sinus seen?
8. Name two radiolucencies seen on the maxillary incisor radiograph.
9. Does the maxilla or the mandible have the denser trabecular pattern?
10. In which area are nutrient canals easiest to identify?

chapter 9 Radiographic interpretation: developmental disturbances of teeth and bone

The inclusion in this text of two chapters on interpretation is not meant to imply that it is the role of the dental auxiliary to make the final radiographic diagnosis. At the present time, the final diagnostic role rests with the dentist. However, to produce adequate diagnostic films the dental auxiliary must know what relevant information is being sought from the radiograph. If one knows how periapical pathologic conditions appear radiographically, one also understands the necessity of seeing the entire periapical area of the tooth in question in order to make a proper diagnosis. If the dental auxiliary knows how difficult, or in some cases impossible it is to interpret caries on radiographs with horizontal overlapping of the teeth, it should motivate the auxiliary to try to avoid this error in technique.

The purpose of Chapters 9 and 10 is to give the dental auxiliary some basic understanding of radiographic interpretation, to stimulate interest, and to show the importance of producing an adequate diagnostic radiograph.

ERUPTION OF TEETH

Periapical radiographs of children below the age of 12 will reveal some evidence of a mixed dentition. The permanent teeth or tooth buds are seen apically to the deciduous teeth they will replace (Fig. 9-1). The first and second permanent molars, which have no deciduous predecessors, can also be seen in various stages of formation (Fig. 9-2). The force of the erupting permanent tooth will cause resorption of the deciduous roots, with resulting loosening and loss of the tooth. If root formation is not complete, a radiolucent area may appear around the root tip. This radiolucency is the dental root sack and should not be confused with periapical pathologic conditions. There is a range (±9 months) in the normal development and eruption time of the dentition. Systemic diseases such as hypopituitarism and hypothyroidism will cause retarded development; other diseases such as cleidocranial dysostosis can cause overretention of the primary teeth and retarded permanent tooth eruption.

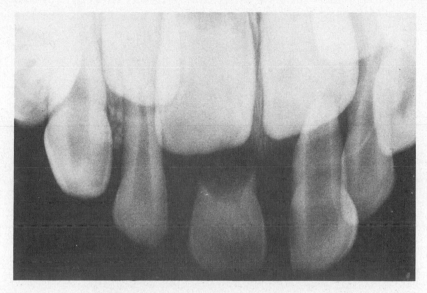

Fig. 9-1. Maxillary central incisor area in child. Permanent teeth are seen in bone. Note root resorption of deciduous central incisor due to eruptive force.

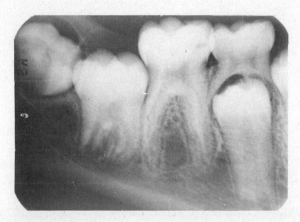

Fig. 9-2. Mandibular mixed dentition. Note incomplete root formation on second premolar, second molar, and developing third molar.

IMPACTED TEETH

The radiograph is the prime diagnostic tool in locating and defining the relative position of the impacted tooth because most impacted teeth are not visible on intraoral examination. The maxillary and mandibular third molars are the most common impactions. These teeth must be localized not only in their vertical position by periapical, panoramic, or lateral oblique films but also in the buccolingual relationship by occlusal films.

Radiographically the bony impaction may be seen completely or partially covered by bone (Fig. 9-3). A soft tissue impaction will not be covered by bone, but in many cases the outline of the covering soft tissue can be seen on the radiograph (Fig. 9-4).

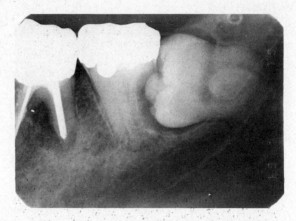

Fig. 9-3. Bony impaction of mandibular third molar. Note relationship of tooth to mandibular canal and root resorption of second molar.

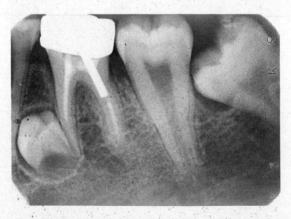

Fig. 9-4. Soft tissue impaction. Note supernumerary tooth in premolar area.

SUPERNUMERARY TEETH

Supernumerary or extra teeth, as well as their relative position to other teeth, are easily detectable on the proper radiographs. As with impacted teeth the buccolingual relationship can be established by the use of occlusal films. The most common supernumerary teeth are mandibular premolars, maxillary incisors, and fourth molars. If the supernumerary tooth occurs between the maxillary central incisors it is called a *mesiodens* (Fig. 9-5). If it is positioned distal to the third molar it can be referred to as a *distodens*. Supernumerary roots can also occur that may or may not be detected radiographically (Fig. 9-6).

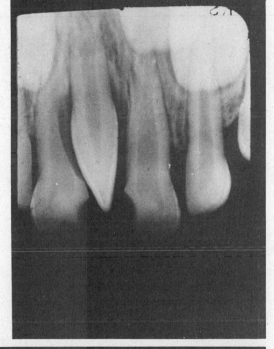

Fig. 9-5. Mesiodens. Supernumerary tooth between the central incisors.

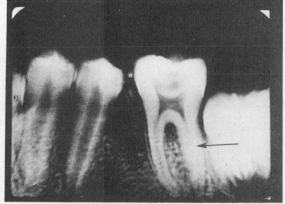

Fig. 9-6. Supernumerary roots. After extraction it was found that there were two distal roots on the first molar. Note how wide distal root is.

CONGENITALLY MISSING TEETH

Anodontia, congenitally missing teeth, is the failure of teeth to develop. It can occur in either the primary or the adult dentition. It can be either a single missing tooth, many missing teeth (oligodontia), or complete anodontia. Anodontia can only be definitively diagnosed by radiographic examination (Fig. 9-7).

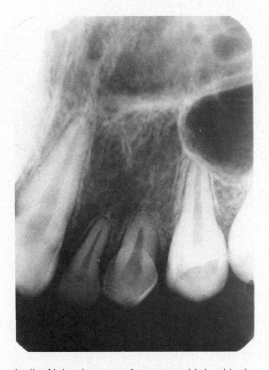

Fig. 9-7. Anodontia. Note absence of permanent lateral incisor and canine.

ENAMEL PEARLS

Enamel pearls, enameloma, are small spherical-shaped pieces of enamel attached to the roots of teeth. They are asymptomatic and are usually discovered through routine radiographic examination.

FUSION

Fusion is a condition that results from the joining of two teeth early in their development. There is usually a single large crown with two root canals (Fig. 9-8).

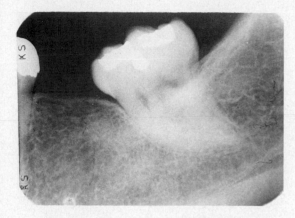

Fig. 9-8. Fusion. Note single crown with two root canals.

GEMINATION

Gemination occurs when a single tooth germ splits during its development. It usually appears as two crowns with a common root canal (Fig. 9-9).

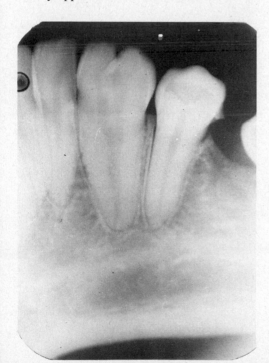

Fig. 9-9. Gemination. Note two crowns with common root canal.

CONCRESCENCE

Concrescence is the joining of two teeth by their cementum.

DENS INVAGINATUS

Dens invaginatus, or dens en dente, is not a "tooth within a tooth" as it is commonly referred to but an invagination of the enamel organ within the body of the tooth. The point of invagination of the enamel is usually the cingulum of the tooth (Fig. 9-10).

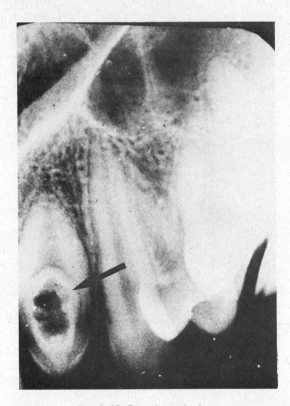

Fig. 9-10. Dens invaginatus.

DILACERATION

Dilaceration is a permanent distortion of the shape and relationship of either the crown or the root of the tooth. It is thought to be caused by trauma during the development of the tooth (Fig. 9-11).

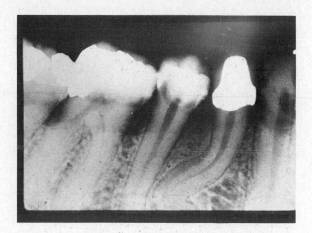

Fig. 9-11. Dilaceration. Note curved root on first premolar.

MALPOSITION OF TEETH

Teeth that do not occupy their normal position in the mouth are said to be malposed. They may be prevented from achieving their normal position by tumors, cysts, supernumerary teeth, or lack of space. If a tooth occupies the normal position of another tooth it is said to be transposed.

TAURODONTIA

Taurodontia is a hereditary disturbance in which the teeth have large crowns and pulp chambers with short roots.

TURNER'S TOOTH

Turner's tooth is a condition in which a permanent tooth has developed under a nonvital deciduous tooth and whose development has been affected by chronic infection. Irregularities in the normal contour and radiolucencies can be seen in the crown of the permanent tooth.

275

FISSURAL CYSTS

Fissural cysts are always found in predictable anatomic locations because they develop along embryonic suture lines. The nasopalatine cyst is seen as a radiolucency in the midline near the apices of the maxillary central incisors. The globulomaxillary cyst is always seen as a pear-shaped radiolucency between the maxillary lateral incisor and canine. The median palatine cyst is seen as an oval radiolucency in the midline of the palate. The nasopalatine and globulomaxillary cysts are seen on periapical films of their respective areas; the median palatine cyst is seen best on occlusal films (Figs. 9-12 to 9-14).

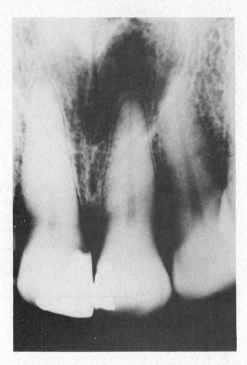

Fig. 9-12. Nasopalatine cyst.

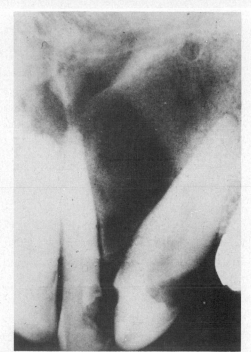

Fig. 9-13. Globulomaxillary cyst.

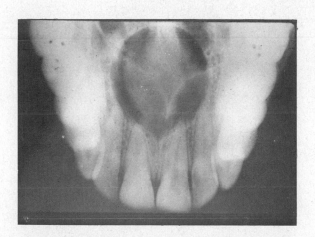

Fig. 9-14. Median palatine cyst seen on occlusal film.

CLEFT PALATE

The failure of embryonic processes to fuse in development causes clefts. These clefts can occur in the hard or soft palate or both. Clefts can disturb the dental lamina and so anodontia, malposition, or supernumerary teeth may result. Radiographically the cleft appears as a continuous radiolucent band (Fig. 9-15).

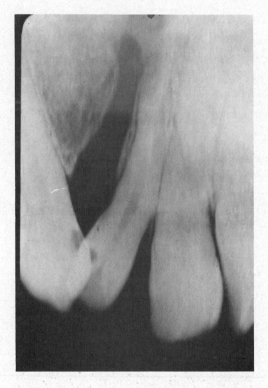

Fig. 9-15. Cleft palate. Note radiolucent defect between lateral incisor and canine.

DENTIGEROUS CYST

A dentigerous cyst forms when the developing tooth bud undergoes cystic degeneration. The cyst may surround or be lateral to the developing tooth. If cystic formation begins from the dental lamina before the tooth bud forms, this is called a *primordial cyst* (Figs. 9-16 and 9-17).

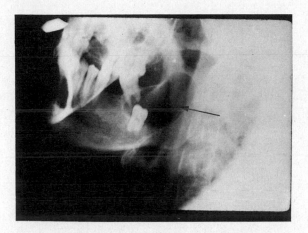

Fig. 9-16. Dentigerous cyst seen on lateral oblique film.

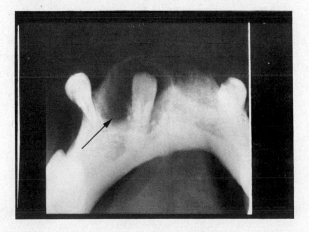

Fig. 9-17. Dentigerous cyst seen on mandibular occlusal film.

STUDY QUESTIONS

1. How can radiographic examination help in evaluating tooth development and eruption?
2. How can supernumerary teeth be detected? Localized?
3. How does an impacted tooth appear radiographically?
4. Distinguish between concrescence and fusion.
5. Describe a dilacerated tooth.
6. How does a cleft palate appear radiographically?
7. What is the best radiographic projection to visualize a median palatal cyst?
8. Distinguish between a nasopalatine cyst and a globulomaxillary cyst in regard to radiographic appearance and location.
9. Describe the radiographic appearance of a dentigerous cyst.
10. Why is it important to localize impacted teeth in three planes?

chapter 10 Radiographic interpretation: caries, periodontal disease, and pulpal, periapical, and bone lesions

CARIES

Detection of caries is probably the most frequent reason for taking dental radiographs. Caries is seen on radiographs as a radiolucency in the crowns and roots of teeth. The caries process is one of decalcification of the hard tooth structure with subsequent destruction. This decrease in density allows greater penetration of the x-rays in the carious area and resultant radiolucency on the film. The degree of radiolucency on a given film will be determined by the extent of the caries in the buccolingual plane in relation to the density of the overlying tooth structure. Radiographic interpretation of caries can be misleading in regard to relative depth and position in the tooth, as well as differentiation from other radiolucencies. Caries will always be farther advanced clinically than the radiographs indicate because the bacterial penetration of the dentinal tubules and early decalcification will not produce significant changes in density to affect the penetration pattern. The depth of the caries in relation to the pulp can also be misleading. Since the radiograph portrays a three-dimensional object in two planes, what may seem to be an obvious pulpal exposure radiographically may be the result of superimposition of images.

Caries that occurs only in the enamel is said to be *incipient* and is difficult to detect radiographically because there has not been any great change in the density of the tooth structure. Most advanced caries involving dentin in either the crown or the root of the tooth will be seen on properly taken radiographs. However, small, deep occlusal, buccal, or lingual carious lesions may not be seen. This is because the decrease in density caused by the caries is small compared with the total buccolingual density of the tooth.

It is in the diagnosis of interproximal decay that radiographs are most important. Interproximal caries is best seen on bite-wing radiographs. If the paralleling technique is used, caries is also seen well and undistorted on periapical films. In the bisecting-angle technique the vertical angulation may distort or even mask interproximal caries. This is especially true of recurrent decay under old restorations. Bite-wing radiographs are also useful in detecting poor contact, fit, and contour of metallic fillings, as well as overhangs and broken fillings (Fig. 10-1).

Horizontal angulation, as mentioned in Chapter 3, is extremely important in caries diagnosis because an overlapped film will not show the interproximal surfaces clearly and therefore will be of no diagnostic value.

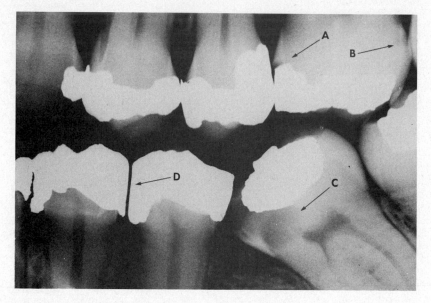

Fig. 10-1. Interproximal caries on bite-wing radiograph: *a,* recurrent; *b,* incipient; *c,* advanced; *d,* open contact.

Occlusal caries

A careful clinical examination with a mouth mirror and an explorer will detect occlusal caries earlier than will radiographic interpretation. The absence of radiographic findings is a result of the superimposition of the dense buccal and lingual cusps on the relatively small carious area in the occlusal fissures. Occlusal caries is not seen radiographically until it has reached the dentoenamel junctions, at which point it appears as a horizontal radiolucent line. As the decay progresses into the dentin it appears as a diffuse radiolucent area with poorly defined borders. This appearance differentiates it from advanced buccal or lingual decay, which has more defined borders (Fig. 10-2).

Very often radiographs of teeth with deep or broad occlusal pits and fissures will show radiolucencies that resemble caries. These normal variants can be differentiated by examination with a mirror and an explorer.

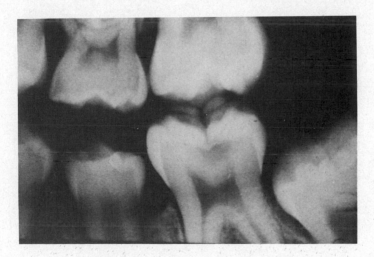

Fig. 10-2. Occlusal caries in mandibular first molar.

Buccal and lingual caries

Early lesions on these surfaces may be very difficult, if not impossible, to detect radiographically because of the superimposition of the densities of normal tooth structures. As the caries progresses the radiolucency is characterized by its well-defined borders. Although it is theoretically possible to differentiate radiographically between buccal and lingual decay on the basis of sharpness of the image, it is not clinically important. The differentiation is done more easily with a mirror and an explorer. It is impossible to judge the relationship of buccal or lingual caries to the pulp on radiographs because the depth of the caries lies in a geometric plane that is not recorded radiographically (Fig. 10-3).

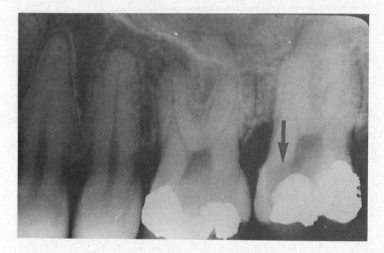

Fig. 10-3. Buccal caries.

Interproximal caries

The first sign of interproximal caries is a notching of the enamel, usually just below the contact point. As the caries progresses inward it assumes a triangular shape with the apex of the triangle toward the dentoenamel junction. As it invades the dentin the caries spreads along the dentoenamel junction and proceeds toward the pulp in a roughly triangular-shaped pattern (Fig. 10-4).

The radiographic appearance of interproximal caries will be affected by the size and shape of the contact of the tooth involved. A tooth with a broad contact point will not show the caries as well as one with a narrow contact point because of the greater density of the tooth structure surrounding the caries (Fig. 10-5).

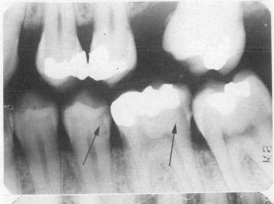

Fig. 10-4. Interproximal caries.

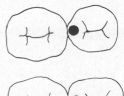

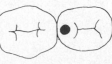

Fig. 10-5. Diagram illustrating effect of contact point on caries interpretation.

285

Conditions resembling caries

There are many radiolucencies seen on dental radiographs that may be mistaken for caries. The final diagnosis of caries is always made by corroborating the clinical examination with the radiographic findings.

Cervical burnout. Cervical burnout appears as a radiolucent band at the necks of the teeth. It is contrasted because the part of the tooth apical to it is covered by bone and hence more radiopaque and the area of the tooth occlusal to it is covered by enamel and is also radiopaque. In addition to these differences in densities caused by enamel and bone, the concave root contours below the cementoenamel junction will appear as radiolucencies. Cervical burnout is most often observed when there has been no loss of the alveolar bone that provides the radiographic contrast. It is seen most often in the mandibular incisors and molars (Fig. 10-6).

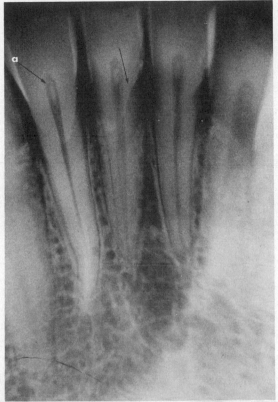

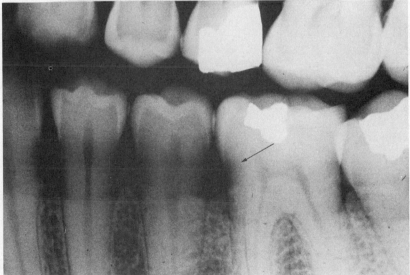

Fig. 10-6. Cervical burnout *(arrows)*. Anterior teeth also show pulp denticles, *a*.

Abrasion and attrition. Radiographically cervical abrasion may resemble caries because it causes a wearing away of root structure and results in a decrease in density in the affected area. The radiolucency produced by the abrasion is usually a well-defined horizontal defect seen at the cementoenamel junction. Evidence of secondary dentin formation and pulp recession in response to the irritant may also be seen radiographically (Fig. 10-7). Attrition, which is defined as occlusal wear on teeth, can be seen clinically and radiographically.

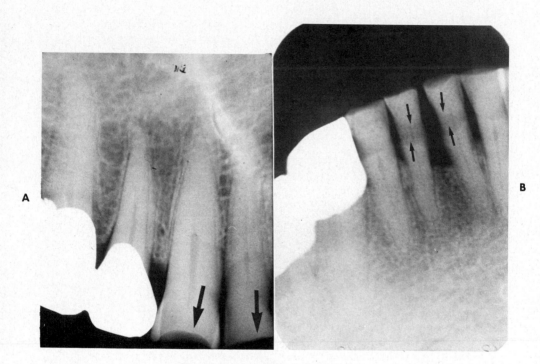

Fig. 10-7. A, Attrition. **B,** Abrasion.

Indirect pulp capping. A radiolucent shadow under a metallic restoration may not always indicate recurrent decay but an indirect pulp capping. In order to avoid a carious pulp exposure in this technique the last remaining portion of decayed tooth is not excavated. A sedative base and permanent restoration are then placed with the hope that secondary dentin will be laid down to protect the pulp. Radiographically the indirect pulp capping procedure will show the radiolucent band of the unexcavated decay near the pulp chamber with a sedative base and permanent restoration (Fig. 10-8).

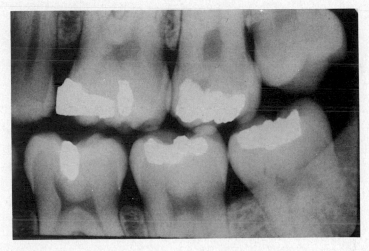

Fig. 10-8. Indirect pulp capping. Note radiolucent area under restoration in maxillary second molar.

Restorative materials. Restorative materials such as silicates, acrylics, and some composites may resemble caries radiographically (see Fig. 8-15). Recently some brands of composite filling material have had radiopaque materials added to their formulation (see Fig. 8-16). Differentiation from caries of the radiolucent filling can be made on the basis of the regular geometric outline of a cavity preparation and the presence of a radiopaque cement base. All base and pulp capping formulations that have a metallic component (for example zinc oxyphosphate, zinc oxide, calcium hydroxide) will appear radiopaque.

PERIODONTAL DISEASE

Periodontal disease has both soft tissue and bone components; there are diagnostic radiographic limitations in both aspects of the disease process. Radiographs should be taken only after clinical examination has detected periodontal disease. The limitations of the radiographs lie in their inability to locate soft tissue margins, the superimpositions of buccal and lingual alveolar bone, overlapped anatomic structures, and variations in the periodontal ligament space.

Even with these limitations radiographs are useful in (1) identifying predisposing factors, (2) discovering early bone changes, (3) approximating the amount of bone loss and location, (4) evaluating the prognosis of the affected teeth, and (5) evaluating post-treatment results.

Predisposing factors

The detection of predisposing factors is one of the most important roles of radiography in periodontal disease. The treatment or prevention of early periodontal disease is much easier and has a higher success rate than efforts made once the disease has progressed farther. The detection and elimination of local irritants are essential steps in prevention or actual periodontal therapy.

Calculus. Both subgingival and supragingival calculus are the most common of all local irritants. Early deposits, small and not fully calcified, will not be seen radiographically. Even when calcified supragingival calculus, which is seen most often on the lingual surface of lower anterior teeth and the buccal surface of upper molars, will not be seen clearly in its early stage because of superimposition of tooth structure (Fig. 10-9). Subgingival calculus on the proximal surfaces is more easily detected in the early calcified stages. The calculus is seen as an irregularly pointed radiopaque projection from the proximal root surfaces (Fig. 10-10).

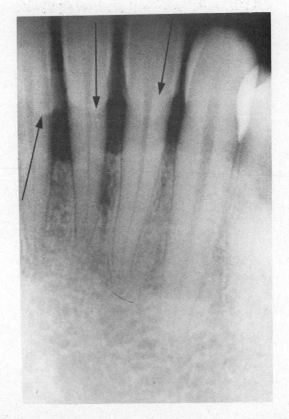

Fig. 10-9. Supragingival calculus on lingual surfaces of lower incisors.

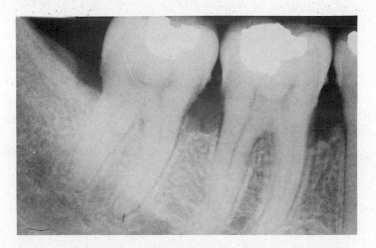

Fig. 10-10. Subgingival calculus. Note bone loss.

Restorations. Radiographic examination will reveal restorations with open contacts, poor contours, overhanging and deficient margins, and caries, all of which are etiologic factors in periodontal disease (Figs. 10-11 to 10-13).

Anatomic configurations. Only through radiographic examination can information about the size, shape, and position of the roots of periodontally involved teeth be obtained. These factors are important in evaluating the present condition and planning periodontal restorative therapy.

The crown-root ratio refers to the length of root surface imbedded in bone compared to the length of the rest of the tooth. The greater the length of the tooth imbedded in bone, the better the prognosis (Fig. 10-14).

Teeth that have anatomically short roots will have a poorer prognosis periodontally than those teeth with long roots. Teeth with bulbous roots will have more area for attachment than those with fine, tapered roots. In multirooted teeth the space between the roots is important; teeth with widely spaced roots have a better periodontal prognosis. Adjoining teeth whose roots are close together have a poorer prognosis than those with adequate areas of interseptal bone.

Gingivitis. There are no radiographic findings of gingivitis other than the presence of local irritants.

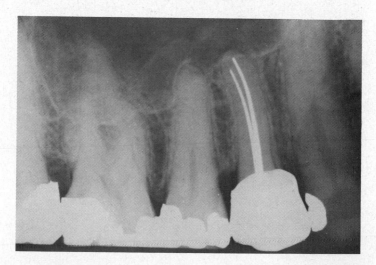

Fig. 10-11. Overcontoured crown and bone response.

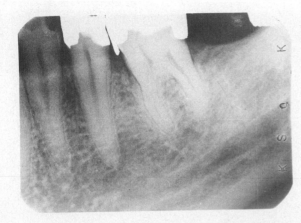

Fig. 10-12. Restoration with open contact and overhang. Note bony response.

Fig. 10-13. Restoration with overhang. Note heavy calculus formation in other areas.

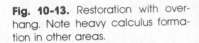
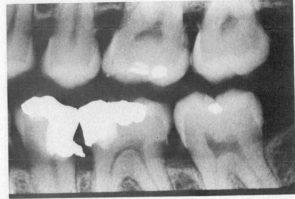

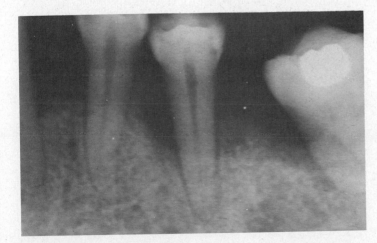

Fig. 10-14. Crown-root ratio — unfavorable.

293

Periodontal changes

Early (Fig. 10-15). This stage of periodontal change is characterized radiographically by changes in the crest of the interproximal bone septum and triangulation of the periodontal membrane. Triangulation is the widening of the periodontal membrane space at the crest of the interproximal septum that gives the appearance of a radiolucent triangle to what is normally a radiolucent band. The normal crest of the interseptal bone runs parallel to a line drawn between cementoenamel junctions on adjoining teeth at a level 1.0 to 1.5 mm below the cementoenamel junction. The crest of the septa will normally have a distinct radiopaque border. Fading of the density of the crest with cup-shaped defects are seen in the early stages of periodontal disease.

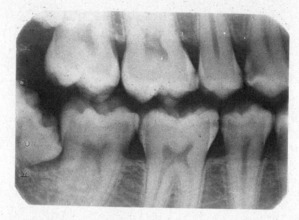

Fig. 10-15. Early periodontal bone loss. Note fading of density of the alveolar crest, slight cupping, and triangulation.

Moderate. In this stage of periodontal change bone loss around the teeth is seen in both the horizontal and the vertical plane. Radiolucencies appear in the furcations of multirooted teeth, indicating bone loss in these critical areas (Fig. 10-16). Horizontal bone loss is resorption that takes place in a plane parallel to a line drawn between the cementoenamel junctions on adjoining teeth (Fig. 10-17). In vertical bone loss the resorption on one tooth root sharing the septum is greater than on the other tooth, the so-called infra-bony pocket (Fig. 10 18). It is in this stage that horizontal bone loss on the buccal or lingual surfaces may go undetected because of superimposition. Careful examination of the radiograph may reveal a difference in density indicating different levels of bone on the buccal and lingual surfaces (Fig. 10-19).

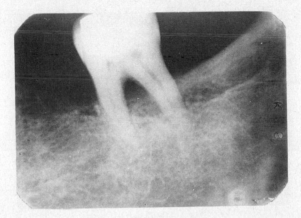

Fig. 10-16. Moderate to advanced bone loss showing bifurcation involvement.

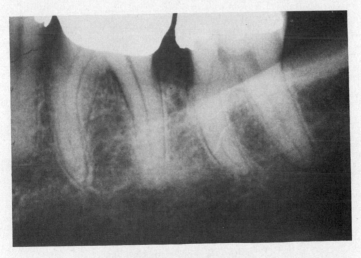

Fig. 10-17. Horizontal bone loss.

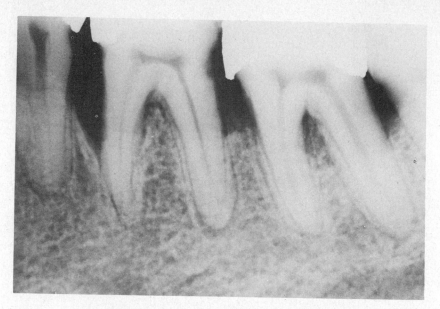

Fig. 10-18. Vertical and horizontal bone loss.

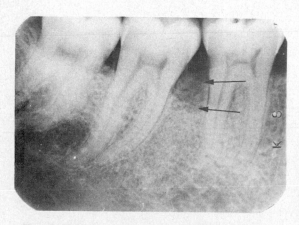

Fig. 10-19. Different levels of buccal and lingual bone as indicated by arrows.

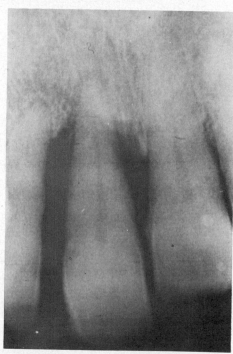

Fig. 10-20. Advanced periodontal bone loss.

Advanced (Fig. 10-20). This stage of periodontal disease is easily identified radiographically by the advanced vertical and horizontal bone loss, furcation involvement, thickened periodontal membranes, and indications of changes in tooth position.

Periodontal abscess (Fig. 10-21)

The radiographic signs of a periodontal abscess vary greatly. In order to make such a diagnosis, there must be an acute clinical manifestation. Periodontal abscess is caused by the occlusion of an existing pocket; therefore the radiograph of the acute episode may not vary greatly from previous films of the existing condition that produced the pocket. In other instances there may be signs of rapid and extensive bone destruction.

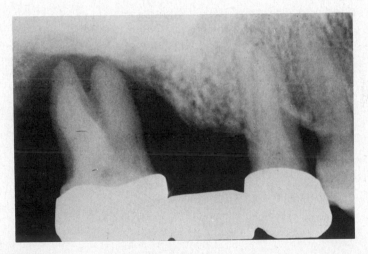

Fig. 10-21. Periodontal abscess. Patient had acute buccal swelling and facial edema.

PULPAL LESIONS

High pulp horns and large pulp chambers can occur in all age groups, not just in the young patients of which these findings are characteristic. The normal size and shape of the pulp chamber and canals change with age, in certain developmental anomalies, and in response to local irritants. Gradual reduction in the size of the pulp chamber and canals accompanies aging. This reduction is marked by the deposition of secondary dentin at the walls of the chamber and canals (Fig. 10-22). Radiographically secondary and regular dentin appear the same and can only be differentiated by the changes in the shape of the chamber and canals that accompanies aging. The formation of secondary dentin with the resulting obliteration or narrowing of the pulp chamber and canals can be caused by different types of irritants. The most common causes are deep caries, pulp capping, deep-seated restorations, attrition, abrasion, and a healed tooth fracture (Fig. 10-23). This decrease in pulp and root chamber size is also seen in the developmental disturbances dentinogenesis imperfecta and dentinal dysplasia (Fig. 10-24).

Pulp stones or calcifications appear as well-defined radiopacities within the pulp chamber (Fig. 10-25). A radiolucent line may be seen separating the stone from the pulpal wall or it may be attached to the floor or wall of the chamber. The stones, which are composed of either dentin or calcified salts, will have the density and appearance of dentin.

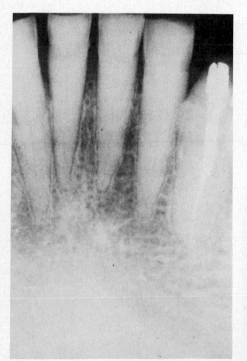

Fig. 10-22. Pulp chambers receded with age. Secondary dentin formation.

Fig. 10-23. Secondary dentin formation in second molar in response to caries and restoration.

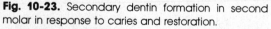
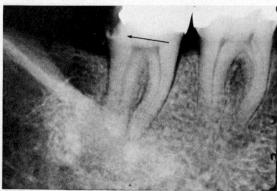

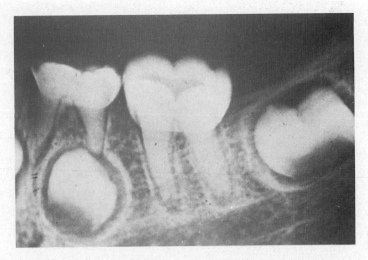

Fig. 10-24. Dentinogenesis imperfecta. Note early calcification of pulp chamber and canals.

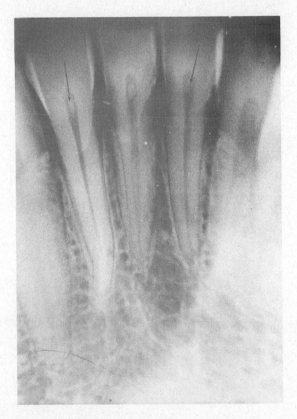

Fig. 10-25. Pulp stones in lower incisors.

Pulpitis

There are no radiographic signs of pulpitis in the pulp chamber. Normal, inflamed, or necrotic pulp all appear the same. The only possible radiographic findings in pulpitis are the causative factors such as caries, pulp exposure, previous pulp capping, or deep restorations (Fig. 10-26). The pulp may vary in radiographic density. This is not because of differences in vitality but because of the differences in object density of the overlying tooth structure.

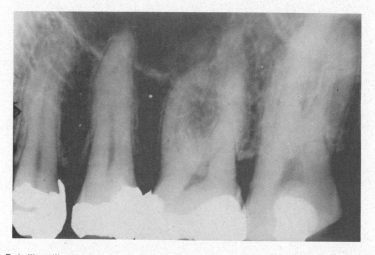

Fig. 10-26. Pulpitis with no apical changes. Second premolar was acutely sensitive to thermal stimulation and was found to be partially nonvital.

PERIAPICAL LESIONS

Periapical lesions are seen in the apical tissues surrounding the tooth after the pulp has become necrotic. The periodontal membrane, lamina dura, and alveolar bone are the affected tissues. This necrosis, or degeneration of the pulp may be a result of carious invasion of the pulp or physical or chemical trauma. The exudate from the pulp first spills into the periodontal ligament, causing a thickening that can be seen radiographically (Fig. 10-27). The pressure then causes resorption of the lamina dura and alveolar bone. At this point, depending on certain factors, a cyst, granuloma, or dental alveolar abscess may develop. It is almost impossible to differentiate radiographically between a periapical cyst and a periapical granuloma (Figs. 10-28 and 10-29). The dentoalveolar abscess may cause root resorption and a more diffuse radiolucency (Fig. 10-30). A fistulous track leading from the abscess to the oral cavity, if present, is very difficult to see on radiographs because of its tortuous course.

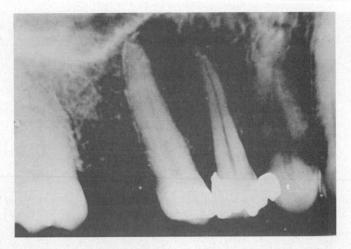

Fig. 10-27. Thickened periodontal membrane on maxillary first premolar caused by pulpal necrosis.

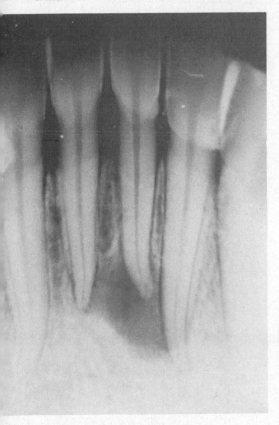

Fig. 10-28. Periapical granuloma.

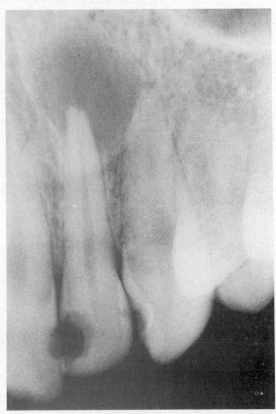

Fig. 10-29. Periapical cyst.

301

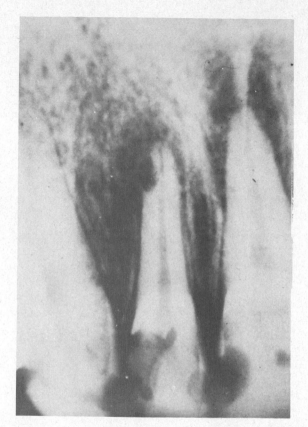

Fig. 10-30. Dentoalveolar abscess.

Periapical condensing osteitis

Periapical condensing osteitis is recognized by the formation of dense bone around the apex of a tooth in response to low-grade pulpal necrosis. This asymptomatic condition is seen most often at the mandibular premolar and molar apices (Fig. 10-31).

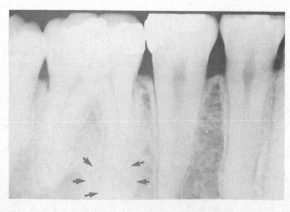

Fig. 10-31. Periapical condensing osteitis in mesial root of first molar.

Residual periapical lesions

Residual periapical lesions are the radiolucent pathologic areas that remain following extraction of the teeth they surrounded if the apical area was not curretted after surgery (Fig. 10-32).

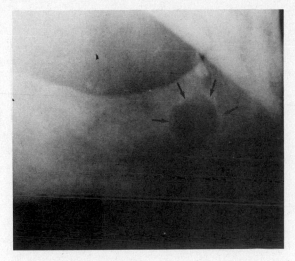

Fig. 10-32. Residual cyst of mandible seen on lateral oblique film.

Hypercementosis

Hypercementosis is a condition characterized by the buildup of cementum on the root of the tooth. Normally it is difficult to distinguish cementum from dentin because of its thin layers. The buildup of cementum makes the root appear "club" shaped instead of its usual conical appearance (Fig. 10-33).

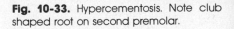
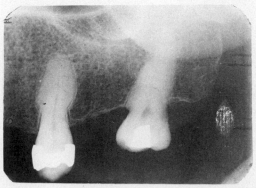

Fig. 10-33. Hypercementosis. Note club shaped root on second premolar.

Root resorption

Root resorption can be caused by chronic infection, trauma, pressure from tumors or cysts, or rapid orthodontic movement (Figs. 10-34 to 10-37).

Internal resorption (Fig. 10-38). The cause of this internally destructive process is unknown. The radiographic findings of internal resorption are irregularities and widening of the usually smooth, tapered outline of the root chamber. In advanced cases the irregular outline of the resorption can be seen reaching the periodontal ligament.

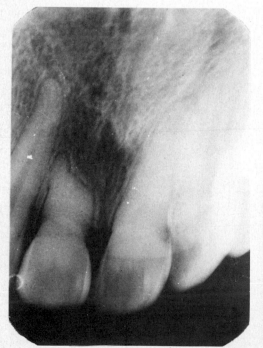

Fig. 10-34. Root resorption resulting from trauma.

Fig. 10-35. Root resorption resulting from chronic periodontal infection.

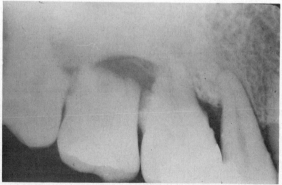

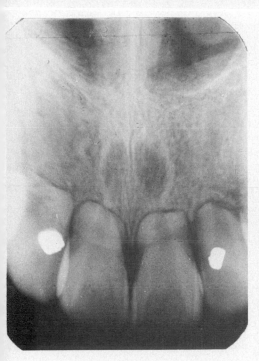

Fig. 10-36. Root resorption resulting from orthodontic movement.

Fig. 10-37. Root resorption resulting from a malignant tumor.

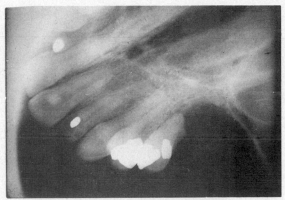

Fig. 10-38. Internal root resorption.

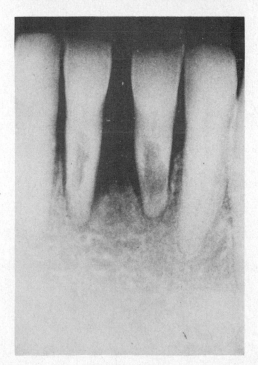

305

External resorption (Fig. 10-39). The cause of this resorptive process is also unknown. Radiographically teeth with external resorption will have a round or oval radiolucency lateral to or superimposed over the pulp canal. If it is superimposed the outline of the normal canal can be seen through the superimposition. If the radiolucency is lateral to the pulp canal it will not, in its early stages, communicate with the pulp canal.

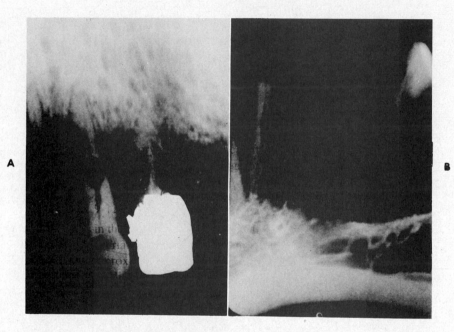

A   B

Fig. 10-39. External root resorption.

Cementoma (fibro-osteoma) (Fig. 10-40)

Cementoma is a three stage lesion that is asymptomatic and self-limiting and for which there is no treatment indicated. It occurs at the apical region and it originates in the periodontal membrane of the tooth. In its first stage it is radiolucent and resembles periapical disease. The second stage is mixed because the radiolucent lesion starts to calcify. In its third stage it is totally radiopaque.

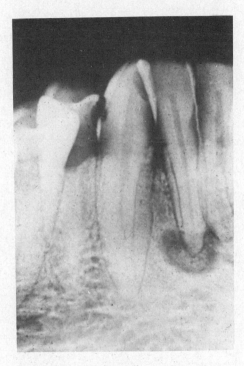

Fig. 10-40. Cementoma; all teeth test vital.

TRAUMATIC INJURIES

Fractures of teeth, especially anterior teeth, are very common. Clinically and radiographically a fracture of the crown of a tooth is easier to detect than a root fracture. The fracture will be seen on the radiograph as a radiolucent line or the missing part of the tooth will be apparent (Fig. 10-41). A root fracture is also seen as a radiolucent line but is much more difficult to visualize because of superimposition of alveolar bone trabeculation (Fig. 10-42). Fractures of the teeth in the vertical axis may not give any radiographic findings.

Fractures of the maxilla and mandible may be seen in part on periapical film but larger views such as panoramic or extraoral are needed for complete visualization (Fig. 10-43).

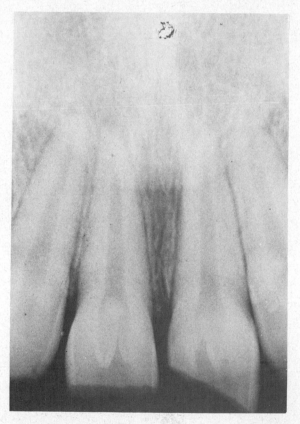

Fig. 10-41. Fractural crowns of maxillary central incisors. Note proximity of fracture lines to pulp chambers.

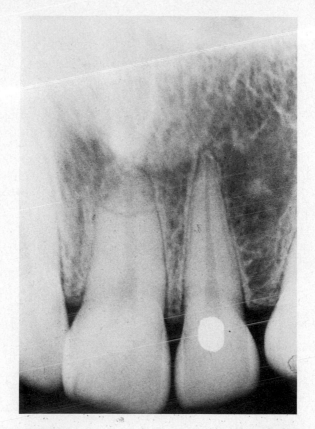

Fig. 10-42. Root fracture of maxillary central incisor.

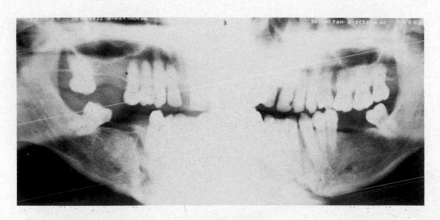

Fig. 10-43. Panoramic radiograph showing fractured mandible.

FOREIGN BODIES AND ROOT TIPS

It is possible to have any sort of foreign body imbedded in the jawbones. Only those that are radiopaque will be seen radiographically. Metallic foreign bodies are the easiest to see and the most common. These radiopacities may be amalgam, burrs, broken instruments, needles, metallic fragments from an external source (Fig. 10-44), or metallic implants (Fig. 10-45).

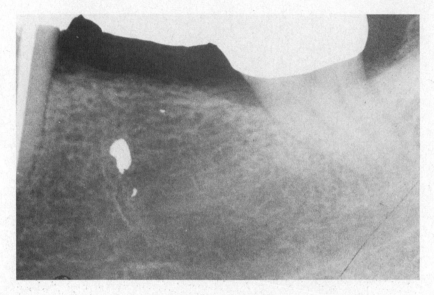

Fig. 10-44. Metallic foreign body in mandible.

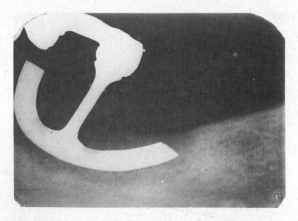

Fig. 10-45. Metallic implant of the mandible serving as distal abutment. Note thinning of bone indicating start of rejection process.

Retained root tips will have the density of tooth structure (Fig. 10-46). It is sometimes very difficult to distinguish between the retained root tip and dense areas of bone. One way to differentiate between the root tip and dense bone areas is the appearance of a pulp canal or the conical shape of a root tip. These root tips should be localized radiographically in three dimensions before surgery is attempted.

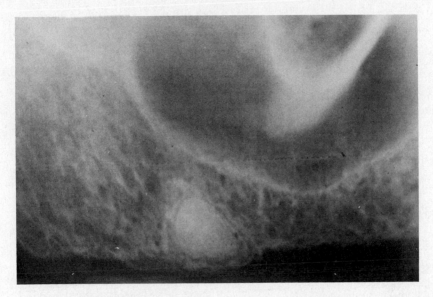

Fig. 10-46. Retained root tip in maxillary molar region.

EXTRACTION SOCKETS

Extraction sockets may be radiographically evident in the bone up to 6 months after surgery. The area eventually fills in with bone in the normal trabecular pattern (Fig. 10-47).

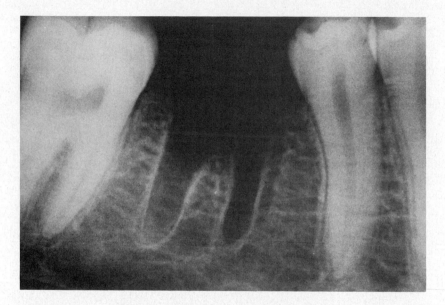

Fig. 10-47. Extraction socket in mandible.

SALIVARY STONES

Salivary gland disease is often treated by the dentist. Although the salivary glands and ducts are soft tissue, radiographs are still important in the diagnostic workup. Salivary stones (sialoliths) are a common cause of obstruction, secondary swelling, and infection. Since the sialolith is calcified it can be detected on radiographs. Stones in the submandibular duct can best be seen on a mandibular occlusal film (Fig. 10-48). A lateral oblique or panoramic film is used when the stone is in or near the neck of the submandibular gland.

For the parotid gland, in which stones are not so common, a lateral oblique, posteroanterior, or soft tissue film placed in the mucobuccal fold can be employed.

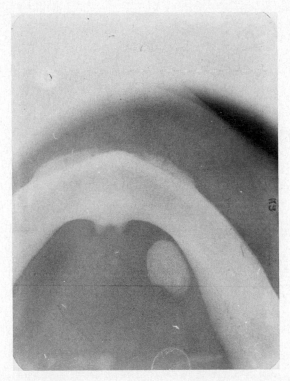

Fig. 10-48. Occlusal radiograph of edentulous mandible showing radiopaque salivary stone in submandibular duct in floor of mouth.

CYSTS AND TUMORS

All cysts located in bone will be seen as radiolucent areas. Tumors can appear either radiolucent or radiopaque. When the cyst and the tumor appear radiolucent it is because the lesion has destroyed normal bone and replaced it with less dense cystic or tumor tissue (Fig. 10-49). If the lesion is radiopaque this signifies that the new tumor tissue being formed has a greater density or size than the tissue it is replacing (Fig. 10-50). Tumors of bone and cartilage will appear radiopaque while all other tumors will appear radiolucent. It is mandatory for the dentist to be able to see the entire lesion before any type of treatment is instituted.

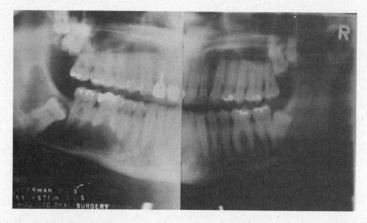

Fig. 10-49. Radiograph of tumor (ameloblastoma) enveloping teeth.

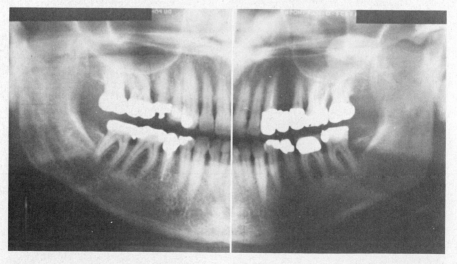

Fig. 10-50. Panoramic radiograph showing well-defined radiopaque tumor in left maxillary sinus. Compare right and left maxillary sinuses.

314

The possibility of malignancy must be explored. In general malignancies tend to have poorly defined radiographic borders and will destroy normal anatomic structures (Fig. 10-51). Benign tumors and cysts will expand slowly with clearly defined borders. Their slow growth tends to displace rather than destroy structures (Fig. 10-52).

In large pathologic areas it will be necessary to use the accessory techniques described in Chapter 5 to visualize the entire lesion and to make a radiographic diagnosis.

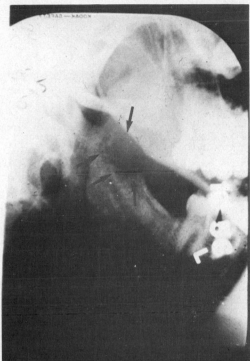

Fig. 10-51. Lateral oblique radiograph showing destruction of coronoid process by malignant tumor.

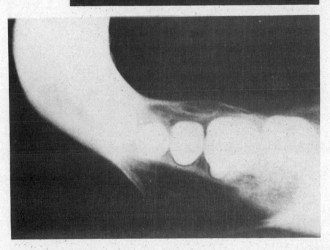

Fig. 10-52. Occlusal radiograph showing expansion of buccal and lingual plates of mandible caused by benign tumor.

STUDY QUESTIONS

1. Why do caries appear radiolucent on radiographs?
2. Name some other conditions found on radiographs that might be misinterpreted as caries.
3. Why is it difficult to visualize occlusal and buccal caries radiographically?
4. Name some predisposing factors to periodontal disease that can be seen on radiographs.
5. Describe the appearance of calculus on a radiograph.
6. What are the radiographic signs of periodontal disease.
7. Differentiate between internal and external idiopathic resorption.
8. Would the bite-wing film be the projection of choice for diagnosis of traumatic injury to teeth? Why?
9. Differentiate between hypercementosis and a cementoma.
10. What characterizes a malignant tumor radiographically?

Glossary

administrative radiographs Radiographs taken for other than diagnostic purposes, for example, radiographs taken for verification for third party payment.

ala-tragus line An imaginary line between the ala of the nose and the tragus of the ear that is kept parallel to the floor for maxillary periapical and bite-wing films.

alternating current (AC) Electric current that travels in one direction and then reverses its flow to go in the opposite direction.

ampere The unit of measurement of the amount of current flowing in an electric circuit. The unit milliampere (mA) is $^1/_{1000}$ of an ampere and is the important unit of current measurement pertaining to an x-ray tube.

Angstrom unit (Å) A unit of measurement equal to $^1/_{100,000,000}$ cm; x-ray wavelengths are expressed in Angstrom units.

anode The positively charged side of the dental x-ray tube. It contains the tungsten target at which the electrons are aimed and from which x-rays are emitted.

atom The basic unit of matter, composed of a positively charged nucleus around which negative electrons revolve.

atomic number The number of protons in the nucleus of an atom. Its symbol is Z and is written as the subscript, for example, $_3$Li.

attenuation Absorbing or weakening of an x-ray beam because of passage through a material.

autotransformer A transformer that has only one coil and a series of taps that allows it to step up or step down voltage.

background radiation The ever-present ionizing radiation in the environment. Its sources are cosmic rays, radioactive materials, and nuclear fallout.

barrier A radiation-absorbing material such as lead, concrete, or plaster used to protect the area from radiation.

becquerel The new unit of radioactivity produced by the disintegration of unstable elements. It is to be phased into use by 1985 and replace the curie.

binding energy The energy expressed in electron volts that binds the orbiting electrons in their respective shell around the nucleus of an atom.

bisecting-angle technique A technique for intraoral periapical radiography where the film packet is positioned as close to tooth and bone as possible and directs the central x-ray vertically at an imaginary line that bisects the angle formed by the long axis of the tooth and the film packet.

bite-wing radiographs Intraoral films that show only the crown portions of opposing teeth in the biting position.

bremsstrahlung The release of a photon of energy by a bombarding electron slowed and bent off course by an atom.

buccal-object rule In localization if the object moves relatively on a second radiograph in the opposite direction as the horizontal tube shift, then the object is bucally positioned.

calcium tungstate The fluorescent material used to coat intensifying screens.

cassette A wrapping or container for x-ray film that is light-tight and will permit penetration of x-rays. Cassettes may be plastic, cardboard, or metal.

cathode The negatively charged side of the dental x-ray tube. It contains the tungsten filament and the molybdenum focusing cup.

cathode ray The stream of electrons in the x-ray tube traveling from filament to target.

central ray That x-ray that is located in the center of the x-ray beam as it leaves the tube head.

cephalometric radiograph The process of measuring the skull by means of radiographs.

317

cervical burnout The shadow seen interproximally on radiographs that is caused by the concavity in the root surface at that area. It may resemble caries.

characteristic x-rays X-rays that are produced when orbiting electrons in an atom fall from outer shells to inner shells after an orbiting electron is knocked out of one of the inner shells by bombarding electron.

chromosomes One of a definite number of rodlike bodies, containing genes, found in the nucleus of a cell. At the time of cell division they divide and distribute evenly in the resulting cells.

collimation The process of restricting the diameter of the x-ray beam.

collimator A device that limits the size of the x-ray beam.

cone The pointed PID on the dental x-ray machine through which the x-rays travel after leaving the tube.

cone cutting The mistake made by not centering the x-ray beam on the film, leading to unexposed areas on the film.

contrast The difference in densities between adjacent areas on the radiograph.

cosmic ray A radiation that has its origin outside of the earth's atmosphere, for example, the sun's rays.

curie The unit of measurement of the number of nuclear disintegrations of a radioactive element. The curie will be replaced by the becquerel by 1985.

cycle of electric current The sine wave plot of the change in polarity of an alternating current circuit where the current travels first in the positive direction and then in the negative direction.

definition or detail The degree of clarity on a radiograph.

density (film) The degree of blackness on a radiograph.

density (object) The relative mass of an object through which the x-ray beam passes, which makes it appear either radiopaque or radiolucent.

developer The solution used in the processing of exposed x-ray film that precipitates silver

from the silver bromide crystals of the film emulsion that have been energized by x-rays.

developer cutoff The blank area on processed radiographs that results from insufficient level of solution in the developer tank in the darkroom.

diaphragm The lead doughnut-shaped collimating device found in the dental x-ray machine that limits the beam size.

dimensional distortion The distortion seen in the bisecting-angle technique when parts of the object farther from the film are foreshortened in relation to parts of the object closer to the film, for example, buccal roots of maxillary molars versus palatal root.

direct current (DC) Electric current that flows in one direction and does not reverse itself.

dose The amount of radiation energy absorbed per unit mass of tissue at a particular site.

dose equivalent A concept that allows for the fact that not all radiations are identical in biologic effects. The dose equivalent is expressed in rems.

duty cycle The number of seconds in a minute that a dental x-ray machine can be operated without overheating.

duty rating The number of consecutive seconds that a dental x-ray machine can be operated before overheating.

electric current The flow of electricity through a circuit.

electromagnetic radiation spectrum A group of energy-bearing invisible radiations whose individual properties are determined by their wavelengths. X-rays are electromagnetic radiations.

electron A negatively charged particle, which is a constituent of every neutral atom.

elongation The distortion on a radiograph that results in lengthening of the image.

emulsion The silver bromide suspension in gelatin that is coated on the x-ray film base.

exposure A measure of the ionization in air produced by x or gamma radiation.

exposure time The amount of time, expressed in seconds or impulses, that x-rays are generated.

extension paralleling technique A technique for intraoral radiography that uses a 16-

inch focal-film distance and film packet placement parallel to the long axis of the teeth and central ray direction perpendicular to both object and film.

extraoral films Radiographs that are taken with the film outside the patient's mouth.

fallout A form of background radiation produced by atomic explosions.

filament The tungsten wire found at the cathode in the x-ray tube, which when heated will boil off electrons.

film badge A recording device worn to record one's exposure to ionizing radiation.

film reversal The improper placement of the film packet in the patient's mouth, which results in an underexposed film with geometric images (herringbone pattern) on it, caused by the useful beam striking the lead foil backing before the film itself.

film speed or sensitivity An expression of how much radiation for what period of time (mA) will be necessary to produce an image on the film.

filter An aluminum disk placed in the path of the useful beam, which absorbs the softer, less penetrating radiations.

fixer The solution used in the processing of exposed x-ray film that removes the unaffected silver bromide crystals from the emulsion.

fluorescence The property of emitting visible light when struck by radiation.

focal-film distance (FFD) The distance from the focal spot (target) at the anode of the dental x-ray tube to the film. It is usually expressed in inches, for example, 8-inch FFD.

focal spot *See* Target.

focal trough That plane of an object that is seen clearly on a laminograph.

fog A detrimental density imparted to radiographic image by the film base and chemical action on unexposed silver grains. Fog is increased by inadvertent exposure to white light or a poor safelight.

foreshortening The distortion on a radiograph that results in shortening of the image.

full-mouth survey A series of intraoral radiographs that gives diagnostic information for all teeth and desired bony areas. It is usually composed of periapical and bite-wing films.

gag reflex The coughing, retching, or vomiting caused by contact of the film packet, holding device, or operator's fingers with the patient's palate or other intraoral tissues.

gamma rays Radiations that emanate from radioactive materials.

gene The basic unit of inheritance located in the chromosome; it determines hereditary characteristics.

genetic effects The changes produced in an individual's genes and chromosomes; usually refers to those changes in reproductive cells.

gray The unit of absorbed dose of radiation that will replace the rad by 1985.

half value layer The thickness of a specific material that attenuates the x-ray beam intensity to one half. It is an expression of beam quality.

horizontal angulation The aiming of the x-ray beam in the horizontal plane.

intensifying screen A coating of fluorescent material on a suitable base that will intensify the radiation, thus permitting a decrease in exposure time. Intensifying screens are usually used with metal cassettes.

inverse-square law An expression of the relationship between the exposure time and the focal-film distance. It states that the intensity of the radiation varies inversely to the square of the distance.

ion An electrically charged (+ or −) particle of matter.

ionization The process by which an electrically stable or neutral atom or molecule gains or loses electrons and thereby acquires either a positive or negative charge.

ionizing radiation The property of radiation that produces ions when interacting with matter.

isotopes Atoms whose nuclei have the same number of protons but a different number of neutrons.

kilovolt One thousand volts.

kilovolt peak (kVp) Used in dental radiology to describe the kilovoltage setting on the control panel. It implies that not all the x-rays generated will be of the penetrating power called for; rather the numerical setting will be the peak.

319

labial mounting A means of mounting and viewing processed radiographs so that the observer is looking into the patient's mouth with the patient's right side on the viewer's left.

laminograph A radiograph of a three-dimensional object that shows a predetermined plane clearly while blurring out all other superimposed structures.

latent image The term used to describe the x-ray film after it has been exposed. The film contains the latent image that will be made visible by the film processing.

latent period The delay between exposure of an organism to radiation and manifestation of change produced by that radiation.

lingual mounting A means of mounting and viewing processed radiographs so that the observer seems to be looking at the teeth from within the patient's mouth with the patient's right side on the viewer's right.

localized exposure The measurement of radiation to the area of the body that is in the path of the direct beam of radiation.

long cone Used to refer to cones on x-ray machines where focal-film distance is 16 inches or greater.

mass number The number of nucleons (protons and neutrons) in the nucleus of an atom.

milliampere (mA) One one-thousandth ($^1/_{1000}$) of an ampere.

milliroentgen (mR) One one-thousandth ($^1/_{1000}$) of a roentgen.

molecule The smallest particle of a substance that retains the properties of the substance.

mutation The chemical effect of a change in a gene or a chromosomal aberration.

neutron A particle that has no charge but has mass, found in the nucleus of an atom.

nucleus The positively charged, relatively heavy inner core of an atom.

object The structure being radiographed, such as tooth or bone.

object-film distance The distance between the object and the x-ray film.

occlusal film A large piece of intraoral film that is placed on the occlusal surfaces of either upper or lower teeth and used to portray objects in the third dimension.

orbit A prescribed path or ring that electrons travel in around the nucleus of an atom.

output The amount of radiation being produced by the x-ray machine. It is measured in roentgens per second.

packet A wrapping or container for intraoral x-ray film that is light-tight and will permit penetration of x-rays. Packets are usually made of paper or cardboard.

panoramic film A radiograph that shows both the mandible and the maxilla in their entirety.

pantomogram A panoramic radiograph taken by using curved surface tomography.

paralleling technique A technique for intraoral periapical radiography where the film packet is positioned parallel to the long axis of the tooth and the central ray is directed perpendicular to both tooth and film packet.

penetration The ability of x-rays to pass through an object and reach the film.

penumbra The amount of unsharpness of the image.

periapical radiograph An intraoral film that shows the entire tooth and surrounding bony structures.

photon A discrete unit of energy.

point of entry Anatomic location on the patient's face at which the central x-ray is aimed so that the x-rays will strike the center of the film in the patient's mouth.

position indicating device (PID) That part of the x-ray machine (cone, rectangle, or cylinder) that aligns the useful beam to the object and film.

primary radiation X-rays coming directly from the target of the x-ray tube.

progeny The descendants of an individual.

proton The positively charged particle that has mass, found in the nucleus of an atom.

quality control (assurance) Programs that assure the quality of radiographs by monitoring the x-ray units, chairside technique, and processing on a predetermined schedule.

radiation The emission and propagation of energy in the forms of waves or particles.

radiation absorbed dose (rad) A unit of absorbed radiation. In dental radiology a rad is approximately equal to a roentgen.

radiation exposure The process of being struck by radiation, either primary or secondary.

radiograph The visual image produced by chemically processing the effects of x-rays on film.

radiolucent The black areas on radiographs.

radiopaque The white areas on radiographs.

receptor The material (film, film screen, or xeroradiographic charged plate) that is affected by the x-ray beam and from which the visible image is formed.

receptor holder The object that holds and positions the receptor (film) in the patient's mouth, for example, a bite block.

rectangular collimation Limiting the shape of an x-ray beam to a rectangle instead of the conventional circle.

rectification The blocking of the flow of current in one direction in an alternating current circuit.

right-angle technique *See* Paralleling technique.

roentgen The basic unit for measuring x-ray (ionizing radiation) exposure in air. It is the amount of radiation needed to produce one electrostatic charge in 1 cubic centimeter of air. The milliroentgen (mR) is $^1/_{1000}$ of a roentgen (R).

roentgen equivalent man (rem) The expression of dose equivalent. The dose of radiation that will produce the same biologic effects in humans as are produced by 1 roentgen of x radiation. For x-rays, the rem equals the rad.

safelight Illumination used in the darkroom that will not affect the film emulsion.

sagittal plane of head A median vertical longitudinal plane that divides the head into right and left halves.

scattered radiation Radiation that, during its passage through a substance, has been deviated in direction. It may also have been modified by an increase in wavelength. It is one form of secondary radiation.

secondary radiation Radiation that comes from any matter being struck by primary radiation. Secondary x-rays are less penetrating than primary x-rays.

selection criteria Those factors that determine whether radiographs are necessary and useful in a specific clinical situation.

shielding Preventing or reducing the passage of radiation particles.

short cone A term used to refer to cones on dental x-ray machines where focal-film distance is 8 inches.

sievert The new unit of dose equivalent that will replace the rem.

sight development An unacceptable technique used to process x-ray films where the time the film stays in the developer is related mined by periodically looking at the developing image under safelight conditions.

silver bromide The x-ray–sensitive crystals that are used in the film emulsion.

soft x-rays X-rays of longer wavelengths that have low penetration.

somatic effects Effects of radiation on all cells except the reproductive cells.

target That part of the anode that the high-speed electrons strike and that produces x-rays and heat. In dental x-ray tubes the target is usually made of tungsten.

thermionic emission effect The production of free electrons by passing an electric current through a tungsten filament and thus heating the filament.

time-temperature development A technique used to process x-ray films where the time the film stays in the developer is related to the temperature of the solution within a stated acceptable temperature range.

tissue sensitivity That scale of sensitivity of various tissues in the body to radiations. Some tissues (for example, epithelium) are very radiosensitive, while others (for example, bone) are relatively radioresistant.

tomography *See* Laminograph.

total body exposure The radiation dosage that reflects the effects on the whole body of the person exposed.

transformer An electric device that can either increase (step up) or decrease (step down) voltage.

useful beam The part of the primary radiation that passes through the diaphragm aperture and filter and exits through the PID.

vertical angulation The angle made between the x-ray beam and a line parallel to the floor.

voltage The difference in potential in an electric circuit. It is this difference that causes the current to flow.

wavelength The distance from the crest of one wave to the crest of the next wave. The length of the wave determines its energy.

xeroradiography An imaging system that uses a charged plate as the receptor. The images are then printed by the xerographic copying process.

x-rays Penetrating electromagnetic radiations having wavelengths shorter than those of visible light, which are produced by bombarding a metal target with high-speed electrons.

Index

A

Abrasion, 288
Abscess
  dentoalveolar, 300, 302
  periodontal, 297
AC; see Alternating current
Accessory radiographic techniques, 133-167
Acetic acid, 200
Acrylics, 242, 289
Aim in using dental x-rays, 52
Air bubbles on film, 225
Ala-tragus line, 78
Alopecia, 53
Alternating current, 10, 11, 21
Aluminum filter, 29
Alveolar bone, 236, 237
  resorption of, 300
Alveolar crest, 236
  fading in density of, 294
Alveolar ridge, 255, 256
Amalgam restorations, 242, 244
Ameloblastoma, 314
American Dental Association, film speed recommendations of, 35, 56
American National Standards Institue, 39
Ampere, 10
Anatomic landmarks, 165
  interpretation of, 235
Anatomy, normal radiographic, 229, 235-266
  of crowns and roots, 234
  of mandible, 254-259
  of maxilla, 246-253
  tooth, 236-237
Angstrom units, 5
Angulation
  horizontal, 81
  negative, 112
  positive, 112
  vertical, 81
    in bisecting technique, 37, 111, 112

Anode of x-ray tube, 14, 21
Anodontia, 272
ANSI; see American National Standards Institute
Anterior nasal spine, 246, 247
Anterior palatine foramen, 263
Anterior restorations, 242, 243-244
Arch, narrow, 178
Articular eminence, 261, 266
Articular fossa, 266
Atom, 5
  lithium, 6
  neutral, 6
  structure of, 6
  tungsten, 20
Atomic number, 6, 23
Attrition of teeth, 288
Automatic film processing units, 212-213
  advantages of, 212
Autotransformer, 10
Auxiliary, dental; see Dental auxiliary

B

Background radiation, 50
Backscatter, reduction of, 32, 34
Beam; see X-ray beams
Becquerel, 46
Bedridden patients, 185
Benign tumors, 315
Bent films, 100-101
Beta particles; see Electrons
Biologic effects of radiation; see Radiation, biologic effects of
Bisecting-angle technique, 36-37, 71 111-132
  advantages of, 111
  with caries, 282
  dimensional distortion of, 72-73
  disadvantages of, 35, 72-73, 112
  elongation in, correcting, 124
  errors in, 96, 124-126
  focal-film distance for, 111, 112